Airfairy, Dragon, and Rockstar

Field Notes on Practicing Medicine in a Pandemic

Melissa Bentley, M.D.

Livingston Press
University of West Alabama

ISBN 13: trade paper 978-1-60489-421-9
ISBN 13: e-book 978-1-60489-422-6

Library of Congress Control Number: 2026946530

Typesetting and page layout: Joe Taylor, Kelly West
Proofreading: Tricia Taylor, Kelly West, Trinity Cates, Kelly Scott, Maggie Smitherman, Savannah Brown, JT May

"The Wild Geese" by Mary Oliver was first published by Atlantic Monthly Press

I heard David Whyte recite his included poems at his wonderful retreat.

Cover Design: Kelly West

This is a work of nonfiction. The stories, essays, impressions, and details are factual, as far as memory can be trusted. To protect privacy, the clinic's name has been changed, the specific tribe is not identified, and the names and distinctive aspects of the histories of individual patients have been changed and shifted about a bit.

Livingston Press is part of The University of West Alabama, and thereby has non-profit status.
Donations are tax-deductible.

Airfairy,

Dragon,

and Rockstar

Field Notes on Practicing Medicine in a Pandemic

Dedication

Dedicated, with deep gratitude, to Dr. Hardy,
to my other teachers, mentors, care team;
to my patients;

To Nature, Art, and Science.
And, of course, to Rockstar.

CONTENTS

Air Fairy I: bloody hands and 100-hour work weeks

Air Fairy isn't really a person. She was named, or called out, by my psychologist, who continues attempted exorcism… so perhaps she is a devil, possessive at times, taking possession of my frame, I mean. But then, I am not sure what she is—I suppose a fairy, Air Fairy, but I do not believe in fairies. Sorry, Tinkerbell, perhaps some readers will clap their hands on your behalf. If I were a Jungian, I might call her a type or complex. I don't know if she is just me, or part of me, or an evil spirit who nonetheless feels, at times, more like a protector or—

I do not know. Maybe a villain—so then she could have an "origin story." Or a superhero, superhuman—since at times it seems Air Fairy-me is selfless, tough, ignores pain, fatigue, hunger, all sorts of wimpiness for self-focus, in order to get things done. To manage, to take care of business.

This will be part of her origin story then. Because this book is about being a doctor, the practice of medicine in a pandemic—how it can be done—with Air Fairy, a Dragon, and a Rockstar—stay tuned. What follows is a sketch, the outlines of A.F., to lay out the dilemma she poses, or the strategic partnership she provides or the… well—something.

Like many demons, perhaps, Air Fairy was likely forged in the furnace of a difficult early childhood. For me, this was a time when illness and the real possibility of death hovered, heavily, always; when it seemed if I needed or complained or grew or wanted too much, I would harm those around me and be left. Air Fairy grew wings to keep me tightly wrapped, early on, then to keep me without needs, a bonsai—small, or even more aptly, an air plant without even the need for space in the soil. To be harmless, move lightly, and as time passed, to be strong. Tough.

From the time I was about five, I wanted to be a gymnast and was finally signed up for tumbling, then for actual gymnastics classes when I was eight. I was so strong. I went to practice initially once a week, then twice, then three times plus Saturdays. I hated to ever miss class, even if I had to walk there and back because no parent was available to take me. Outside of gym time, I did work on my own, upper and lower body training, stretching, and flexibility.

By junior high, I could beat any boy (or girl, but that wasn't impressive) in an arm wrestle. I could do 30 pull-ups, never-ending push-ups. My favorite event was the uneven bars. When I made the team, it was because of the bars. We used chalk and leather "grips"—straps of leather with two or three finger holes at the top and Velcro straps to secure them around the wrists—to keep our hands from sticking as we swung our bodies up onto, or around the bars, to release one and grab the other, or grab nothing and flip in the air.

But even with chalk and grips, hands, skin, palms tear. Children with torn hands cry and want to stop doing further damage, rest from the practice. Theoretical children. Not young Air Fairy, not disciplined, trained gymnasts. So . . .

"Let's see your hands," a coach would say.

Hands would be shown. If terrible open sores, band-aids would be provided. Some girls did not get back on the bars. Would opt for "circuit" which meant endless crunches, push-ups, etc., or sitting in splits, unless that was not challenging, as it was not for the more flexible girls. Then it was sitting in splits with each leg elevated, to extend beyond 180 degrees, sinking the pelvis down between.

My hands split open. Over and over again, blisters across the palms formed, then broke open, then the raw skin beneath scraped off, over-and-over, around-and-around the bars.

My grips were bloodstained. The head coach noticed. I did not cry and did not ask to sit out. "Melissa, come over." I did.

"Could you take off your grips a moment? Show us your hands."

I did.

"Wow, impressive. Great work. Hey, look at this!" Another coach came over. She was not really ever a fan of me. I was not pretty enough and had bad posture and wasn't fun or funny, the way her favorite girls were. But even so, she gave me a little pat on the back, and seemed—dare I say?—a tiny bit tender.

"Do you need a band-aid?" she asked.

It seemed almost as though she was tempting me. Be weak. Show your weakness, your destiny to fail, your need for help.

"I'm okay, thank you for offering, could I go back to bar practice?" If I can be tough, I can keep training, be loved, not harmful, not weak, not needy—an Air Fairy.

The esteem in their eyes strengthened my resolve through the next half hour, until practice ended. It wasn't that I loved pain, I just wanted to be able to manage. I loved the smell of chalk and the taste of sweat in my mouth—and knowing I could do hard things. I could manage and be okay whatever was happening to or around me, or whatever I needed to do. If I cried or stopped—then—then wimp. Just blistered bloody hands. Nothing deadly or dangerous or really harmful. So why cry and . . .

And soon, hands were callus tough. Strength of mind, focus, do what is needed.

About a year after making the team, I fell off the balance beam. Food for Air Fairy. By then, I had advanced some levels, and was doing back flips on the beam, which was terrifying—or would be, but I refused to be afraid. Or tried not to be. Just needed more practice. Air Fairy. No fear, no needs. In doing a dismount one evening, my foot landed between mats. And my foot was stuck, and I fell over. And was ashamed to have fallen, and . . .

"Melissa, what happened to that landing? You were fine, why didn't you stick it? Do you know how many points the judge can deduct for a landing like that?" a coach hollered.

"Sorry," I said. It was hard to talk. It was all I could do to breathe, as I tried somehow to pretend there was nothing really wrong, that I was being a wimp, that the unbearable throbbing in my ankle was nothing, that I could stand it, and stand on it, move it, if I just stopped being dramatic and got on with things.

"Get back up there and do it 20 times perfectly. In a row. Start over if you step out of the landing. Your body needs to learn how to do it right, and your mind can't be afraid."

I nodded.

"Did you hear?" she asked from across the gym.

"Yes, sorry, okay, sounds good," I said, summoning sound from somewhere inside and managing to produce audible words that I hoped came across as at least nearly normal.

I tried. My ankle would not cooperate. It hurt, which was one thing, but it also wouldn't hold me up, or move, it wouldn't "joint," if that is a verb—I tried for ten minutes, twenty, hoping that practice time would run out and that I would not gain coaches' attention in the meantime, just hold on—

Finally, I did show that there was a problem. I think I made a sort of cry/pained/frustrated sound, and a teammate spoke up for me, pointed me out to a coach. This was rare, usually we did not communicate during practice, or show sign of noticing each other. "Melissa, can you come over here?" he called.

I tried to hurry over as I normally would. But couldn't. I limped.

"Are you okay?" he asked.

"Am fine. Just turned my ankle a little, sorry about that. Should teach me to stick landings, right?" I tried to joke.

"Well. Practice is pretty much done, go ahead and call it a night," he said.

I couldn't walk home. I had to call my mom. Fortunately, she was not working, and ultimately we decided to go to an urgent care, where I learned the ankle was broken into several pieces. It was casted and then booted.

No way to practice now. Which was, in a way, horrible, as being a gymnast was a way—a major way—that I could feel okay, strong, able to face anything. I swam and did a stationary bike on my own, every spare minute, and did strength training and flexibility exercises endlessly in the gym. And I was so praised. Any time one of the girls had an injury or complaint, a coach would point out,

"Melissa finished beam practice with a broken ankle, are you not that tough?" I was so proud.

*   *   *

I am no longer a gymnast. But Air Fairy is amazingly adaptable, shape-shifting, phase-shifting, facing and banishing pain, weakness, wimpiness, the familiar foes, whatever the guise. Including a pandemic. Surely it is possible to call another patient, to read another article, to listen to another webinar, if there is any chance at all I might learn something about COVID-19 that will help me help a patient not die? How could I consider going home to sleep, eat—what selfishness, laziness. At work, I stand—partly because it is healthier, and keeps me attentive; and my clinic is generous and bought me an adjustable standing desk. Also, after brain surgery (stay tuned)—this has been invaluable to properly position my head, neck, back, particularly through the telehealth pandemic. But also, sometimes, my legs are really tired. But that is wimpiness. Air Fairy recognizes that. No need to sit. Dangerous, slippery slope to more laziness, wimpy…

Air Fairy was invaluable in medical school and residency. Sleep was weak. And not really an option much of the time anyway. The ACGME had just instituted work-hour restrictions, and our program was dinged if we recorded more than 80 hours of work in a week. (Eighty hours!). But, as our program director pointed out, training, getting a degree/certification from a program that was under review or poorly-regarded, or lost accreditation would hardly be to our advantage. So no one recorded the actual hours worked, easily over 100. There was so much to do and learn, and I feared missing something, doing harm. How could I rest, given that? I arrived early, pre-rounded on patients, worked into the evening, then on call days I spent the night, a shift of thirty hours.

And yet, I loved medicine. Love it. And the feeling of working hard. Being tired because I was working hard. I needed to be tougher.

One of my first nights of overnight call, I was assigned to the CCU, the coronary critical care unit. I saw a patient who had undergone an a-fib ablation—a procedure in which a laser is used to treat areas of the heart that have abnormal electrical activity, atrial fibrillation, in hopes of restoring the normal pace and rhythm. This patient was bleeding: the nurse had noted his blood pressure dropping, called me, and as I approached the bed, I saw blood coming out of his mouth, maybe his nose—it was hard to tell, the dark red fluid was aggressively suctioned by the nurses, the plastic container containing the suctioned blood already half-full. How much blood was that?

A major vessel and his esophagus had been burned through, I learned later. I should somehow have known this as a possible complication of the procedure, though I scarcely knew what "a-fib" was, vaguely knew treatment options… And I did remember that there is a risk of stroke, these patients are on blood thinners to avoid clot formation in the irregularly beating heart. So they bleed. And he bled. A lot. Nothing in the textbook, at least nothing in my mind then, told me what to do with this, bleeding, stroke, clot. Middle-of-night-exhaustion.

The nurses were brilliant and needed nothing from me, really. I asked them to please page the fellow and the attending cardiologist, STAT—I knew I did not know what to do and things were bad and I knew the word STAT—but didn't know what to do. It seemed to take forever for anyone else to arrive. And even as this man lost his blood pressure, and I tried to order whatever the nurses needed…even as he died, I felt myself falling asleep. I was so very tired. And horrified at myself. That I could be sleepy, falling asleep while this man, my patient—though I hadn't actually met him, I was responsible for him, and he was dying, horribly, coughing/choking blood. That is the sort of situation for which Air Fairy was required. One should not be falling asleep when one's patient is dying. And one should study more and know what to do. Or I should anyway. I did not let myself sit. When it seemed I was falling asleep standing, I paced, looking for the help to come, the supremely skilled fellow, the code team, even the always suit-and-tied, well-dressed and cologne-laden attending. Someone, anyone. If I kept moving I could keep awake, maybe think of something, be tough, help, not fail.

A few months later, I was on a surgery rotation at the VA, a challenging site: an ancient building, with the most wonderful patients, with the most horrifying illnesses. When on my General Surgery rotation, I would check the enormous whiteboard Operating Room schedule each morning to see what cases I was to attend, which surgeon I'd be working with, which room, what time.

My first case to "assist" was a vascular surgery and was booked for ten hours. It had indeed taken ten hours. I held retractors and tried not to contaminate the field or irritate anybody or be in the way and maybe, just maybe, do something helpful. I tried to learn: anatomy, surgery, skills, toughness. Channel Air Fairy. By the end, I was utterly exhausted. During surgeries, I could not eat or even drink anything, because then I would have to urinate—and ungown and glove and scrub in and do all of the procedures for sterility again, and waste supplies—when really I was not worth the resources. And maybe I would also miss learning something crucial. And it was about the patient, for heaven's sake, such self-focus. Standing and learning never killed anyone, it was a privilege.

A new day, look at the white board. Another vascular surgery. Deep breaths. A privilege. I saw that the patient was one of relatively few women in the VA system at the time, she was to undergo possible stenting—a major abdominal artery had an aneurysm, and another was full of thrombus—clot. But after the first cuts, we found that her abdomen was full of fluid. This was due to ovarian cancer, widely metastatic; she had lesions and carcinomatous fluid throughout her abdomen and pelvis.

Which should be, and was, devastating. Even with the best care, she would almost certainly die, her abdomen swelling more and more, the cancer spreading—slowed perhaps by surgery, chemotherapy and radiation, but unlikely to be slowed by much—and in the meantime the treatment itself would be horrible for her. But what I felt, if I was brutally honest, was relief. Just relief that the surgery was canceled. There was no reason to stent an aneurysm to keep it from rupturing in the next few years: by that time she would have almost certainly died of the cancer. On the off chance she did have aneurysmal rupture, she might take it as a blessing, an easier way to die. Or so the surgeons said.

So—canceled. Or done after only the first incision, really. And I would be moved to a simple, short gall bladder. Of course I did not want the patient to have terminal, horrible cancer. But I had never met her, as was often the case in this rotation. She was a name and a diagnosis/procedure. Not really my patient, it seemed and… and I was a wimp. Again, horrified at myself. Again, Air Fairy, "You should NOT be tired." I had nothing wrong with me—focus on what needs to be done, work, work harder, learn, be tougher. I decided to read about each case in the medical record before surgeries, to humanize, make the cases into people, so that I did not have this coldness, selfishness. This meant I slept an hour less, ran an hour earlier, got to the hospital an hour earlier, checked the whiteboard an hour earlier. And if I had had a very late night or was on call overnight, and hadn't slept at all, that made it easier, no need for an alarm to wake up, just stay up. Air Fairy.

* * *

To be able to manage, to avoid giving in to sleep, hunger, laziness. As a gymnast, as a resident in training. And now, as a physician caring for vulnerable patients, trying to keep them alive during a pandemic.

A new or newly problematic virus was killing people and there was, is, always more to learn, to read. What masks are protective? Do masks work in the first place? Then, should everyone be wearing them or were they not needed for general public? Soap and water?

Who is at risk? Should I stop ACE inhibitors in patients with high blood pressure, should I start famotidine or fluvoxamine, are vaccines safe, how many cases today, how many beds does the hospital have, do they need an internist who is quite rusty on ICU care, how much can I remember/relearn—to manage a ventilator, do I need to shower every day when I get home and wash my clothes or does that waste water and time, which patients are highest risk, what treatment works, what is the government doing, what is my clinic doing, is that best practice? Endless. New facts, wrong information, and all of it life-threatening or life-saving—but only if I managed to read and learn—not if I was self-focused.

"Bloody hands," Dr. Hardy, my psychologist, said sadly, shaking his head, his white-gray hair shiny, his kind blue eyes cast down. It became a familiar refrain. I developed an abscess in my jaw. My oral surgeon would see me, they had emergency COVID protocols and precautions. But if I took time to do that—what about my patients? I would miss seeing them. Then I might miss doing something that would have helped, even if just one more time advising of the need for distancing—yes, your grandchildren may kill you—or no, a mask will not work if it is worn below your nose...

"I'm on an antibiotic now," I told Dr. Hardy. "It is a stupid mouth infection, it isn't a deadly virus, and as long as I can be tough, not focus on pain and self—then it doesn't matter."

"Air Fairy, with bloody hands," he replied.

Untouchables

Untouchable: a word used in the past for a person, particularly a person from India, who belonged to the social group that was considered the lowest. This word is now considered offensive. —from *Cambridge Dictionary*.

As I drive into secure parking, beneath the warehouse-like brick building in which my clinic is located, I marvel, not for the first time, that the large, nondescript square structure contains the color, emotion. and struggle to live that I witness each day. Certain patients, many, are unforgettable. Some days I recall aspects of their ailments. Other days, patient-characters waft in-and-out like ghosts, but friendly, usually, harmless, usually. Immigration and Customs Enforcement Services (ICE) is located on the third floor of our building, downtown. We are across the street from the Department of Workforce Services (DWS) and a methadone clinic. Next-door is one of the three homeless shelters in the greater Salt Lake City area. And we are, of course, on tribal land: in fact the clinic is owned by one of the Native Utah tribes, and any profit goes to them. We are primarily a Medicaid clinic, but see some patients with traditional Medicare, and AIAN—American Indian-Alaskan-Native—patients can come for free. These details may explain the rich diversity, and the poverty, of the patients I see.

It was vitally important to remain open for in-person visits during the COVID-19 pandemic. Homelessness, refugee status, mental illness made virtual appointments difficult or impossible, while also making regular care crucial. Fortunately, through Indian Health connections, we were able to obtain PPE, personal protective equipment, in particular N95 masks, as well as gloves and gowns, when these resources were otherwise scarce.

Today, as I take off my new too-cool-for-middle-aged-internist sunglasses, Santana floats into my mind. We were in a strange sort of in-between time in the pandemic, not a surge in cases, but a lot of COVID out there in the community, especially, it seemed, amongst the homeless. And Santana was amongst them, homeless, or unhoused, or "experiencing homelessness" may be the preferred term.

"Good morning, Santana," I said, calling him by his first name, his preference. He always wore large very dark sunglasses. He looked very cool. But was generally hot. Literally. He had hyperthyroidism, which revved up his internal thermostat and other body systems. And he did not reliably take medication to control it, and he did reliably miss appointments. I would get him scheduled with radiology, endocrinology, surgery—to try to further evaluate the cause and possibly treat the condition more definitively. Like so many of my homeless patients—well, housed patients as well—he struggled with mental illness, possible psychosis. The appropriate DSM diagnosis, if there was one, as well as much of his past medical, psychiatric and social history, was unclear, or at least I did not know it. He probably used drugs of various sorts at various times.

"Hi, Doc," he said in his Rolling Stone, slightly hoarse voice. Maybe due to smoking. Maybe his large thyroid was compressing his airway. I hoped not. Of course. Not only did I fear it was compressing his throat, but it was making his heart race, his blood pressure high, causing him to lose weight, suffer anxiety and insomnia. Bipolar disorder was a diagnosis entered into his chart at some point; it was probably or possibly accurate, but how to tell with the hormone problem? This particular day, while I focused, again, on his abnormal thyroid and was giving him another lecture for not taking his medicine and not following up with appointments, he seemed perhaps more fidgety than usual. He squirmed. He was concerned about worms in his rectum.

Santana: “Doc, I’ve got worms, I’m going crazy with itching and pain, I went to the ER it was so bad.”

Me: “Did you go to your endocrine appointment for your thyroid?”

Santana: “No one called me for it. Or I don’t have a phone now. Anyway. There’s something wrong down there.”

Me: “Okay, let’s have a look.”

I step out a moment and put on a better mask and glasses and gloves and ask Nora, my medical assistant, to look up the ER records and to see if she can sweet-talk the endocrinology office into scheduling Santana, again—and to let them know he may not have a phone. Then I knock on the door, and Santana makes a noise that sounds like it is okay to enter, I hope, so I do.

After asking if it’s okay, I have him bend at the waist slightly while I look at his problem.

He does indeed have a very sore-appearing anal region, red and cracked and—and there are worms. They look like wispy bits of white cotton thread, but are almost certainly Enterobius vermicularis or “pin-worms.”

Me: “You have worms.”

Santana: “I know.” With an exasperated, though not unkind, sigh.

I get a dose of albendazole from the pharmacy and tell him to come back in two weeks for his second dose and for me to re-check, and that Nora will give him the new endocrine appointment and he must go to it, again conveying my concerns about his thyroid.

"You can stop at the pharmacy on your way out, they should have a cream for you to pick up—to help with the itching and a refill of the medicine to treat your thyroid problem," I tell him.

"Thanks, Doc," he says. "No one ever looked."

Which is kind of him to say, thanking me. He had told me the problem, his concern, chief complaint, and given the diagnosis—worms. I vaguely remember him complaining before about his "butt itching at night"—how long ago was that? How long has he been suffering with this while I worried about COVID or his racing heart or sky-high blood pressure or chastised him for missing appointments? I look at the records Nora brought, thanking her. He had 3 urgent care visits and an ER visit, and in none of them was a rectal exam performed. Was this because of the pandemic, physical contact carrying heightened infectious risk? Or the psychiatric diagnoses in his chart? Or the patient's chief complaint being lost in the process of obtaining and being distracted by vital signs and labs? Do mental illness, homelessness, and a pandemic render patients untouchable?

I see another patient in person in clinic, Fnu, a middle-aged woman who appears old: kyphosis and arthritis bending her bones. She is carrying a purple-and-silver cane, and as always is impeccably neat. Today, her jacket, eye shadow, ironed skirt, polished shoes are matching purple-silver colored. I only recently learned Fnu is not really her name. She is a refugee from Afghanistan, and the visa document that was created when she arrived moved her first name to her last name, and put Fnu—or FNU—First Name Unknown—for her first name. For two years I have called her Fnu—thinking that I was likely mispronouncing it, and feeling some chagrin about that, but never knowing it wasn't her name at all. We are working to correct it, but in my mind she is still Fnu.

I will work to correct that as well.

She has diabetes and high blood pressure, and because she also has coronary artery disease with stents in her heart and compromised kidney function, it is crucial that her blood sugar and blood pressure are well-controlled. If not, she risks a major cardiovascular event, a heart attack or stroke, or further damaging her kidneys to the point that she would need dialysis. Unfortunately, today—through Fnu's daughter and an interpreter—I learn that she has stopped taking her medications. Again. She felt one was making her sick and then just decided to stop all of them, because she wasn't sure which was the problem. Rather than restarting one at a time, she just stayed off all of them, and today tells me that her sister bought her something over-the-counter that covers it all in one tablet a day. Plus one more if needed. She would like me to order those. Her daughter has a cell phone photo, which she brings out and says the words, "Centrum Silver." Then a second photo, Osteo-bi-flex. How I would love to order her the vitamins in a rainbow labeled bottle, and have it make her well.

She did not bring her blood pressure or blood sugar record. Her blood pressure and her hemoglobin A1c are both well-above goal range. Dangerously high. Before beginning a treatment discussion—perhaps stalling to come up with compassion and strategy and words—I listen to her heart. She is sitting on the exam table and my head with stethoscope in my ears is near her chest.

She puts both arms around me and hugs me to her, and says something. The interpreter says "I love you. I mean, she loves you."

Sometimes in medicine, a white coat feels like an invisibility cloak, of sorts. Not that I disappear in it, but I become Dr. Bentley. Which is right. In a chaotic clinic with sick patients, in a pandemic, my sole focus and role is as a doctor, their doctor, caring for them. Caring about them, but professional: not lost in grief, not overwhelmed by the severity of illnesses and the frustrations of the health care system. And not thinking about my own struggles, or anything else, simply a white-coated doctor, focused, aloof by necessity. But this moment with "Fnu"... As a doctor I was, am, an untouchable of a sort. Only she touched me.

And another patient, here in clinic. As time passes, it seems more patients become virtual, or just don't come in—the pandemic worsens, and it seems more precious and dangerous each time I see a patient, in person. This person is Ashley. A woman who struggled for a long time with methamphetamine addiction and was now homeless. She had been in a car accident and injured her back and leg, had had surgery, been put on opiates, then taken off, then found heroin, then found a methadone clinic, and Medicaid, and then started seeing me. She usually has a list of concerns in a notebook in her purse, issues to address at her visits with me. Nora tells me, "She has no complaints, just refill of albuterol inhaler."

It is only when I am in the exam room that she gets her glittery powder-blue purse out from under the hard chair, and pulls out a hot-pink spiral bound notebook and pen. Her list, saved for me...

"Any other concerns?" I ask, thirty-five minutes into her appointment, trying not to have a tone in my voice that indicated anything other than interest and care and desire to help.

"So sorry," she said, which made me fear I had failed with the tone. She looks at her list.

"My feet," she said.

"Is something wrong with them?" I ask. Concern. Care. Feet matter.

"Well, really the left foot, it just really hurts sometimes so that I can't walk," she says, quietly.

"Oh, I am sorry. How did you get here? Let me take a look," I say. No tone, or only of care.

"It isn't too bad today, but sometimes I can't walk," she replies.

I sanitize my hands and adjust my mask and glasses and put her foot up on the stool, cautiously. The skin is cracked and dry, peeling a bit at the heels, but otherwise I don't note anything obviously wrong, the foot itself, the bones and ligaments, the structure seems intact. To my horror, when I look up at Ashley, she is crying, silently.

"Oh, I am so sorry," I say. "Is it so painful?"

She shakes her head. "I can't believe you are touching my foot. It is so disgusting. I am so disgusting. I don't know when anyone last touched my foot."

I would like to fully place blame on the pandemic, but there is the old joke from med school or medicine residency: "How do you hide something from an intern? Put it inside the patient's gown." True enough. How often I do not look, do not hear the patient's "chief complaint," look at my watch rather than a rectum, a foot... And in an honest moment I admit to myself that this has little to do with infectious risks, with COVID.

I x-ray Ashley's foot in clinic. A radiologist will view the films remotely and report them officially, but usually I can see if there is an obvious, displaced fracture. I don't see anything glaring, but get her a walking boot so that she can wear it when it hurts to walk. And then I wrap both her feet in pink, calamine-and-zinc-impregnated compressive wraps, and I order a tube of cream from the pharmacy—not the same cream as for Santana's anal itching, but something to help with the dry cracked skin—and then schedule her to see podiatry. Try to arrange transportation.

I tell Dragon, my dictation device, the bare bones regarding these and other patient "encounters" for the day. Sometimes, I imagine an enormous, scaled creature, responding to my "wake up" command with a fiery yawn, a smoky snort—rather than a microphone icon on my task bar that changes from its "sleeping" horizontal red state to its vertical green state, ready to listen. And I imagine myself a true storyteller, recounting a saga—not a tired doctor speaking into head-gear in an otherwise empty clinic.

It is necessary, of course, to chart, for billing, records, and so on. But also, I think telling the stories is an attempt to preserve them, these moments with these people, as a doctor, working, touching, being with, attending to... It feels hard to pull myself away, leave the fraught sanctuary of clinic. I can feel the exact spot where Fnu's arms wrapped around me, like a purple-silver scarf, as I take off my white coat and leave for home.

Spiders and Skin Peels

"Spiders," says my psychologist, Dr. Hardy.

It is code, or shorthand, a kinder way to indicate delusion—that I am being delusional/psychotic.

I make a sort of sigh/harrumph/self-disgusted noise, and say, under my breath, "I was not the one with spiders in my rectum."

"You were. Are," he says. "Your unconscious mind was trying to be kind to you, and not directly point fingers."

"Does the unconscious have fingers?" I ask. He gives me a finger. The finger. Perhaps a bit of explanation. It was a dream I had, some time ago, in which a patient complained of spiders in her rectum. I did not see them. My thought was that I had this dream because of a patient I had seen recently, who felt he had worms in his rectum. Just a variation on a theme, in the dream. Dr. Hardy helped me see that the likely helpful, "true" interpretation was—is—that I do not see my own craziness. That I avoid looking at or recognizing the crazy thoughts, the sickness inside myself and then that sort of self-distortion leads me to fear I am harmful or doing something wrong or too large—or something. It made sense when he said it, now I'm lost again… fragments of insight, fragments of dreams remembered.

Another dream: I am peeling my skin. Sometimes it comes off in large pieces, which to me feels so very satisfying, like peeling flaking itchy skin off after a sunburn; or peeling back, removing, old wallpaper; or peeling a very thin-skinned tangerine all in one piece. And then I eat the skin. In the dream.

"You are eating yourself," says Dr. Hardy.

"It was a dream," I say. "And only the skin. Only the peeled skin."

"Eating yourself alive," he says.

"It was so satisfying," I say. "Getting the big sheets of skin, peeling. Not eating them. That's sort of disgusting. Like chewing fingernails or dry fingertips or—like eating skin."

I do not think I had a patient with sunburn or pica or something similar prior to this dream. I did have a patient with very dry skin on her feet. Ashley. A woman who struggled for a long time with methamphetamine addiction and was now homeless. See last essay for her story. Many of my patients who use heroin have terrible skin infections. One homeless man was raped in the showers at the shelter, and now will not shower. He had layers of—dirt?—maybe, best case—but layers of stuff that washed off, very satisfyingly.

How lucky, or maybe blessed or—something—I am. To be able to help skin heal, to order salves, to treat rectal worms, or spiders, to bandage and medicate and care. And yet… and yet, for myself—spiders, skin-peels…

*   *   *

I have a disease for which I receive monthly IV infusions of immunoglobulins, a necessary protein, usually produced by the bone marrow. It is needed for fighting off or preventing infection. In my case, in addition to that, the treatment helps with sores: without the treatment, I develop an increasing number of sores on my fingers, sometimes up to my arms, that do not heal, and are, though small, sometimes quite painful—to me. My infusion has been delayed for weeks, maybe a month now. I also don't feel as strong. But that pain and weakness just seem like complaining. And such a minor problem compared to what so many of my patients suffer. I do not really need the infusions, I think, or maybe could do them less often without serious consequences. The treatment is expensive and takes time to do, sometimes as long as four hours, depending on the amount the immunologist orders. That means the nurse and MA at the infusion center are stuck there with me; so much time, so many resources. Wrong of me to take and need so much. Sometimes I am the last patient there, and with my work, the best, or only day that I have enough time free to schedule the treatment is Sunday. That seems wrong too, to be impacting those lives, taking their time, their Sabbath. And yet, if I am not tough enough to ignore the painful sores, to keep going with the fatigue, if I am not careful enough to avoid infection, then I am not able to help my patients.

The reason for the delay is, as might be guessed, the health care system. My administrators decided to change health insurance plans, a fact of which somehow I didn't get notified or in any case was not aware. Until I received a letter from the prior plan that indicated I had no coverage with them—and had not since the first of the preceding month. Confusingly, in that month I had received a new card from them—the original/current health plan. And I also had received messages through their patient portal indicating that they had paid new claims they received. With the new plan, the IVIG treatment required a new prior authorization. I made calls and sent emails, to insurance, to the pharmacy which provides the infusion (which is separate from the infusion center—which I also called). And to my HR department. To my immunologist's office. I left messages, I waited to be transferred to a different department or person, I was "okay being put on a brief hold" for twenty minutes, with being called back. I received one phone call, from the pharmacy. After two weeks.

They needed new "clinicals" since the last they had were from 2020.

This made little, if any, sense to me. The agent, Nicole, who was calling, said that I might have to see my doctor. I had seen her within the last month, I said, and before that—well a few months before that and ... could Nicole possibly try talking to Jamie, my doctor's office manager? He is excellent and should be able to get her the "clinicals." I suppose that means office notes, laboratory data, proof of sufficiently severe disease? In a week—or closer to two—Nicole called again, letting me know that she was able to get this information and had it all submitted as priority, so should hear back in up to fifteen business days... She seemed very proud of this. And it probably was a lot of work. I thanked her.

And the last phone call from the infusion center: approval not yet through, possibly all submitted... and they have the drug, but can't guarantee it is covered, so rescheduled, will postpone a week.

Again.

And I am a physician. And am fine. What do patients without medical knowledge and lacking all ability to navigate all this—how do they manage? So. A need for Air Fairy, to get through days of clinic with sores and minor infections and weakness—to be tough, not wimp, not even a person really—just tough, a doctor. Peel off the person. Ignore the spiders. Be grateful, should not need care anyway, be fine, am fine. And not.

Fighting for Breath

As virus spreads, pandemic rages,
I try to keep my
patients alive.
They cough, run out of air. Then, on air,
over—and—over, this:
a man says, "I can't breathe,"
with his neck beneath
a knee.
He is Black and he dies.

And I am caught,
driving home: surrounded
by rage. Protesters with signs
and cries I support,
but inside
my car, I am terrified
and sigh relief, for police
make a space, hold a line.

That night a new lock-down—

two threats—violence and virus.

I hike with my dog, try to get high, climb, try to see
the city, survey
the damage, to breathe.
There's a fire,
I can see,
it looks close to my clinic.
I perch, watch, hear
news through my headphones:
a police car was toppled, ignited,
and I—
I pet my pup, who is nervous, try
for calm hands, to smile.

I am an essential worker.
I go to work in a lockdown,
through violence or virus.
Shattered glass greets me,
front doors broken, windows smashed.
A black rock sits on the sterile white paper,
the exam room table.
I sweep up glass and mask
my face and work.

The day ends at last, a last

patient cries

on my shoulder.

She is Black.

She apologizes for the damage,

then for crying

mascara on my white coat.

I tell her it is okay.

I listen to her heart,

I listen to her breathe.

I ask about her blood pressure— high—her menstruation—heavy,
painful

her sleep—elusive, troubled.

I lock up, walk her out.

She is the one shielding me.

* * *

Or, Air Fairy commands, "take less space." So I cut out anything nonessential (and also some essential bits? 0% body fat, no excess, but too lean?) So this...

Fighting for Breath

Virus spreads, pandemic rages,

Patients cough, can't breathe, die.

Then a man says

"I can't breathe," His neck under a knee.

That night a new lock-down,

Two threats: violence, virus.

There's a fire, from the foothills,

it looks close to my clinic.

At work I find shattered glass.

A rock on the exam room table paper.

Sweep, mask, work.

A Black patient cries,

apologizes: for the damage,

for crying mascara on my coat.

I tell her it's okay,

listen to her heart, breath, breathe.

The Ethics Prize: Hope, Revised.

"Wake up," I say to Dragon. And pause.

"Go to sleep." Silently, I apologize to my inanimate dictation device—for the unnecessary bother, the uncertainty. Apologies to objects lacking any possible feeling began early—pre-kindergarten, pre-preschool. If I noticed a particular crayon had not been used as much as others, I felt sorry, tried to use it more so it didn't feel left out. Or, at other times, if it seemed I had used one in particular more than the others, so that it was worn down, I was sure to give it some time to rest, use it less…

But back to this day, starting dictation and stopping—apologizing to my dictation device, waking it up, only to put it off. I am not ready to dictate, not settled, not sure. Unlike so much of my life, what I do in clinic—decisions, recommendations, actions related to patients—almost always, somehow… well, the perpetual self-doubt isn't there. I am not me, I am a doctor in a white coat focusing on a patient. All the parts of me that "do" internal medicine work together and just work. It is difficult or impossible for me to describe or explain this well, I realize. I am not an *I* in it. I know my patients, each one, their past and present illnesses, but not just that; I know their stories. I care. And I went to school forever, and I read and gain experience and learn from others. And then I can help. Heal. Solve problems, be my patient's doctor. This very particular patient, my patient.

But today I feel uneasy, unsure. I roll my shoulders and sort of stretch, look around my office. My walls are hung with diplomas, the

Hippocratic Oath, a Nature Conservancy calendar, some paintings done by patients. Plus a corner for Rockstar's agility ribbons. On my bookshelves, I have medical books and Mary Oliver poetry books and the very small proud shelf with journals containing my Thrombotic Thrombocytopenic Purpura (TTP) research articles, a textbook with a chapter I wrote, and a copy of the research poster I presented in Boston and Atlanta. There is a model of a chest cavity, heart and lungs perpetually leaping out and then requiring reassembly, like a toddler's puzzle. There is a plastinated brain, a skull, a vertebral column, another vertebra model that opens out to show the density of the bones: two of them side by side, one healthy, the other osteoporotic. There are abalone shells from my several escapes to Mendocino, them I use as dishes. They hold my reflex hammer, neuropathy mono-filament, and rings and beads and pins from patients—from the tribe, from the displaced, from the Middle East, from Eastern Europe.

Near a copy of my medical license, I have a framed certificate to which I turn now, seeking reassurance or insight, perhaps. It names me, Melissa J. Bentley, M.D., as the recipient of the Medical Ethics Prize, in 2006. It may be the first certificate I received with "M.D." at the end of my name—I would graduate that year. If only, I think now, if only this award meant that what I did was always right. That my ethics in the practice of medicine was unimpeachable, my decisions exact, integrous… right. Unfortunately, it doesn't mean this. It was awarded during our Medical Ethics course to the senior medical student with the best essay on an ethical topic. The prize was $100—which may be a small amount, but it came without stipulations, it was a gift: not a loan, no repayment, no interest rate. The essay was also published in a periodical, *Medical Ethics in Utah*, published by the University of Utah and Intermountain Health Care. They included my picture and that of another prize winner. We both hold plaques and are surrounded by our teachers. I look very small and earnest.

I turn back to the computer. I should start my dictations, get to work, Air Fairy after me for wasting time... but my thoughts still wander. Uncertainty still resides inside my chest cavity. I wonder if my organs will leap out, heart and lungs, like my model.

I feel lucky, still, to have an office. When I first agreed to be a doctor here at this clinic, working for the Tribe, one of their stipulations was that there would be no offices. This struck me as fairly bizarre, but Chris, the office manager at my prior "normal" clinic practice, who had left to help get the Tribe's clinic started, told me that this seemed to them to be symbolically important. And he hoped could be reconsidered with time, but for now—no office. Before Chris took over, an initial group of administrators or owners—business people of some sort—took advantage of the Tribe, or the Indian Health Service (IHS)—or Medicare or Medicaid or some combination of these. They gave themselves tickets to sporting events, lavish lunches, and took the largest, lightest rooms in the warehouse/clinic as their own private offices. I don't know precise details, but clearly the principle to "First Do No Harm" was not followed.

Though the medical assistants, the PA and NP at the clinic used cubicle areas to access computers, or brought laptops with them into patient exam rooms, neither of these options worked for me. I continue to resist having technology between me and my patient in the exam room. No computer, no screens. I hand-write notes for both of us on a paper I have printed out which also has a list of the patient's current medications (usually I pray it is at least close to accurate—an ongoing difficulty). If the list is very long, I write on the backside, otherwise I write below the medicine list—numbered items, our concerns, our plan.

When I am done listening to and examining the patient and drafting this plan, I leave the room and dash to the MAs' desk. I give them the paper plan, which they will scan in for my later time with Dragon, and then they have a copy to give the patient. I tell the MA verbally as well, what is needed, and I hurry into my office to enter orders into my computer for labs, referrals, medications, vaccinations, x-rays, follow-up appointment, etc. It may seem inefficient, but it is a system that I have used for years, and patients and MAs both have said they feel it helps them know the plan, and they like it. For me, it is a double check, the scanned document, not missing something. And importantly to me, it is a way to be sure I am looking at my patient, and not my computer screen. I am talking to my patient and not my computer—the Dragon talk comes later, and then I have to have a private place to dictate. I cannot do that with anyone listening—it is both a violation of patient's privacy, and an impossibility for me.

The solution for the first months (years?) was to commandeer a patient exam room. It was across the hall from the pharmacy, a convenient location, quick consults or clarification face-to-face with the pharmacist—but it was not a very user-friendly office space. At all. My laptop was on the counter near the sink, which leaked/dripped, and I constantly feared ruining my computer. I had no place to sit, really, as there was no place for my legs if I pulled a stool up to the sink/drain/counter. The height of the counter was too low for me to stand, though this is what I did, trying to work my quads, glutes by squatting, or I could spread my legs a bit wide. I tried to do this rather than hunch my back. Hunching over, unfortunately, was my usual busy-clinic-need-to-get-orders-in default posture.

Chris was right, however, and with time—and I hope seeing my dedication and lack of desire for sporting events or catered meals, or other inappropriate use of their money—the tribe converted an exam room into an office for me. Simple, no windows—but four walls, a desk, chair, bookshelves. After I had brain surgery, they even put in a desk with adjustable height, and a computer with two large screens, which made it much easier, less strainful, after removal of bone from my skull and cervical vertebrae and severing of neck muscles and ligaments. Easier to do telehealth during the pandemic, as well, to see and use multiple screens at once without undue strain on my neck. Only important if I was in wimpy mode, Air Fairy points out, if I was focused on myself and not my patients, if I was so weak as to have pain interfere with my work.

But now—I have an office. And a wall with the Ethics Prize certificate. And I return to thoughts about Ethics. The pandemic has presented new dilemmas. As I look about the office, I am avoiding the box on the corner of my desk. It contains five N95 masks, which are to last me the week. They are not "fit-tested" as we were taught necessary in medical school. That has gone by the wayside with the pandemic. They cover the lower part of my eyes, not the right fit.

When it first became clear that simple masks were ineffective in stopping the spread of COVID, N95 masks became impossible to procure. I tried ordering online, and after an exhaustive search, ordered 2 for $80 plus shipping. There were many online scams, but mine did arrive, 3 weeks later. I tried to make my own masks using vacuum cleaner filters and rubber bands. A disaster. I asked my friend, Michael, who is a hospitalist, if he happened to have one, and he said he had a mask he used for working with toxic paints, fumes, cement drilling in his garage, but it was dirty. He himself used a PAPR—a Powered Air-Purifying Respirator—which has a hood, battery pack—looks sort of like a space suit an astronaut would wear. There was some concern that while these protect the wearer they may allow for spread of disease to others—but with proper decontamination and donning and doffing protocols, that seems unlikely. Michael did not think he could get me a PAPR, they cost a small fortune, and I wouldn't have the batteries, the fit testing… But he did give me the industrial N95 mask. I brought him some Tylenol—he couldn't find any, and I had it. We made the exchange in the parking lot while he charged his Tesla downtown, placing packages on car hoods—mine for him the Tylenol, his for me the N95 mask—then waving. I wondered if we looked like we were exchanging drugs.

Fortunately, and, well, amazingly, within a few weeks of learning the importance of a respirator such as an N95 mask, my clinic had them. The IHS somehow managed to keep us supplied with PPE, personal protective equipment, and also, when they became available, with COVID tests and—the godsend—COVID vaccinations. Although I was always cautious in ordering tests, and in using gloves, gowns, face shields, I never didn't have—or I guess I mean I always had—what I needed. Our test turn-around time was always as fast as anywhere in the state, maybe the nation, and results were reliable. We have an excellent laboratory, staff and director, we have supplies from the tribe, transported to my clinic sometimes by private vehicle from the reservation three hours away, to which the IHS had delivered them. Once, Lindy, the lab director at the time, came to me exhausted and relieved, having made this drive on a hot day with dry ice and coolers stacked on her back seats, bringing those precious vials of vaccine.

I felt a familiar mix of astonishment, gratitude, and guilt, undeserving of the resources so many were lacking. But I wanted to work, to help my patients. The N95 masks, then, were precious. And I was going to keep two, then take the box with three remaining to a former colleague, Kathy, after work. I could easily use just two masks for the week, then they would issue me another five. It seemed any virus would not last long on the masks, and I could leave them out in the sun if I was exposed to COVID. The UV rays would decontaminate them. I chewed gum while I worked in the masks, so the inside smelled fresh. The only visible soiling was usually a tiny bit of olive #1 face powder inside the nose piece, from my attempt to conceal a perpetually red nose. It was silly, under the mask of course no one could see it, but a habit, I guess, and a vanity.

My friend Kathy is in her late seventies and had retired, except for her hospice work. She had a handful of employees, a nurse, secretary, CNA, accountant. And she had several dozen frail old patients, whom she saw in their homes, their nursing homes, or their hospital rooms. She had no N95 masks or PAPRs. She had tried to get some online, but was less fortunate: no masks, significant money paid. She would not stop seeing her patients—people who were isolated and lonely at the best of times—and, during the pandemic, appallingly so.

So, I would start giving her a few masks, as often as I could. Were they mine to give? Should I ask if I could? What if I was told no, as I thought was likely? The ethics prize . . . if only . . .

The essay I wrote was, "Some Thoughts on Honesty and Hope." That day during the pandemic, questioning myself endlessly, I wanted to find it. The essay. It seemed important. I think I wanted some evidence that, though it wasn't really a prize for being very ethical—that I was—*ethical*—or at least not too terrible—or something. Every week, every day maybe, new dilemmas. I told my MAs that vaccination, when it became available, was required. They had to get it in order to be allowed to work. I told them this even though the clinic administration didn't mandate it. I fail to see the logic behind not requiring it—maybe political, maybe fear that critically needed staff would fail to come to work? The Tribe's chairman wanted it to be mandatory. But the clinic medical director and administration prevented a mandate. Sadly, the chairman would die within months—of cardiac arrest and heart failure, thought to be related to COVID 19 infection.

Neither of my medical assistants took issue with getting vaccinated. But what if they had?

Or this: I order things from Amazon. I use Amazon Smiles, to make a donation to the Utah Physicians for a Health Environment. I try to order things in a way that they can be delivered all at once, combining deliveries, and I try to support small businesses with the little house icon, and to find ethical, sustainable, harm-free products and companies. But I save myself from having to go into stores, from possible exposure to the virus, while requiring someone else to do potentially hazardous work in a factory, in transport, in delivery.

Or, daily, my drive home after work, to my beautiful old home on sycamore-lined Laird Avenue, with my beautiful Aussie, Rockstar, and my piano, art, books, closet of clean clothes, cupboards containing almonds and fiber cereal, refrigerator with blueberries and yogurt. On my way home, I will have passed tent homes, shopping carts that seem to be full of garbage that are actually belongings, other shopping carts that have a can or two of soup and a huge bag of dog food, a dog bowl, see a muddy-legged Chihuahua chained to the wheels of a cart. I have filled out forms to try to help patients become citizens, patients who have fled war and horror in their home countries, who are homeless in their way too. I see them, I work among or for them—and then I leave. Does my home environment make it possible for me to continue my work through the pandemic, the fear, with a deadly virus I do not understand, with people who are poor, addicted, sick, in need of every sort of help? Or is that an excuse for my daily escape?

I tried to find the Ethics Prize essay on Google. Tried and failed. In 2006, perhaps not everything was published online, even my eloquent, earth-shattering philosophical writing. Ha. I did find something that led me to the University of Utah Archives, and I emailed an archivist, who, it seems, is brilliant, and within minutes, he had emailed me back a PDF—the "Medical Ethics in Utah" Vol 17, Issue 7 from July 2006. The first page of the volume was headed SOME THOUGHTS ON HONESTY AND HOPE—which, of course, was the title of my essay.

The archivist then emailed me again to say he realized that I was the author of the piece. I emailed him that he was brilliant to have found it, thank you.

I confess, I read it with some hesitancy, fearing how juvenile, naïve, and badly-written it must have been. In truth, it seems researched, articulate, and while certainly more optimistic and decisive than anything I could imagine writing today, I was a little impressed with myself. Particularly so since I know I was in the midst of brutal days on the wards, trying to learn all I could and not kill patients or myself in the process. I am so thin in the photo.

I started the essay with a quote, Emily Dickinson, "Hope is the thing with feathers/That perches in the soul." And then write about Honesty: as doctors, with patients; and Hope: as doctors, with patients… I quote Jerome Groopman from "The Anatomy of Hope: How People Prevail in the Face of Illness," in which he describes research showing that—now quoting my own essay—"belief and expectation can block a patient's perception of pain by releasing natural forms of morphine—endorphins and enkaphalins, in hopeful patients." He also relates research related to the consequences of a patient's emotional state on functions of the autonomic nervous system, including heart rate, blood pressure and respiration. These functions impact a patient's illness and response to treatment. "Fear, pain, and emotional distress… make breathing more difficult; furthermore, studies have shown that there is a correlation between hopefulness and recovery." And so on. I end with Some Conclusions, about true and false hope; I mention my mentor, an oncologist with whom I saw patients during my first year of medical school, John Ward. He often said, "Hope for the best, and prepare for the worst."

I conclude, "I have heard and read this mantra in discussions of the best way to approach delivery of distressing findings to patients, and picture this seasoned oncologist seeking out a path for real hope with each patient and then walking with him, turning or backtracking as needed. And beyond this, I have decided that it is okay to allow patients to hope for a miraculous cure, to even hope for that oneself as a practicing, fully aware physician. To simultaneously uphold honesty, the key is to realize that such a cure would indeed, be miraculous—it is not to be expected, but may be a common hope."

Well said, what? But. What then is honesty? What if there is a virus which makes things unclear? What if in the course of a day, the best one can do is try not to fall apart, to keep masked and sanitized, to learn as much as I can, to see the next patient virtually, and the next in person, to give my best guess or relay the best information available—and possibly to be wrong, or to miss something or…?

And hope. Before COVID, my patients were sick, complicated, my clinic often chaotic. In pandemic, it is all of these, we are all of these, still, plus there is a deadly virus circulating, and it is my job to keep them well, alive—all of them, all of us. I have no hope for miraculous cures. An effective vaccine is wonderful, appropriate masks, PPE, resources are incredibly helpful, and the research that has been ongoing in the midst of a pandemic amazes me. But when—well if—the pandemic ends, my patients will be still be poor, refugees, still face discrimination, lack of healthy food, still struggle with addiction, live lives of despair. I can learn as much as I can, share as much as I can, prescribe, teach, love. But cure?

Silver Flask

Felix looked grey. No, actually, he looked sort of silver. Skin, hair, nails.

"Good morning," I said. "How are you?"

We have both been vaccinated, he unmasks with my okay. I leave my mask on.

His teeth shone silvery, smiling, his blue eyes sparkled, as he replied, "Swell, doc. Swelling all over."

It was true. He had both inflammatory arthritis and lymphoma, which meant periodic episodes of synovitis—swelling of the joints, excessive synovial fluid, filling the synovial capsules, leading to warmth, erythema, and swelling; as well as enlarged lymph nodes, in his case primarily those of his neck, posterior cervical, supraclavicular, some in his armpits as well, axillary chains.

When first I saw him, I asked what he used for his arthritis. He was seen in the VA medical system, which was helpful when I had a clinic there, as I did through residency. Though the patient was able to see me at my current clinic using his Medicare, he continued to see specialists, including rheumatologists, at the VA. I was glad, as certain specialists—notably rheumatologists—are few and far between, and I knew several of them at the VA and had great respect for them—their expertise and their care of patients—having in fact rotated through with them for a time. However, though the electronic health record system at the VA is wonderful, and allowed me to see their notes, all of the patients medications, imaging, hospitalizations—when I was working there—outside of that system it is nearly impossible to get this information.

So, fortunately, Felix was sharp as a tack—a silver tack—and could give me a list. Smiling, after reciting his immune system dampening methotrexate and Humira, his occasional anti-inflammatory celexocib or burst of prednisone he said, " But the most effective, Doc, is the WD-40."

I swallowed. "You take WD-40 for your joints?" I ask. "I do feel glad that you have something helpful, but I am not sure that is safe..."

He guffawed. "I only use it topically," he clarified. "Along with the topical lidocaine and diclofenac, and the pills and shot, but it works better than anything, really."

I hoped that very little would be absorbed systemically. I had no idea, and sort of didn't want to know. I so wanted him not to have pain, and he had suffered. Osteoarthritis from his time in Vietnam, jumping in and out of tanks, squatting in the jungle, and who knows what health effects he suffered from Agent Orange and other toxic exposures there. Maybe his lymphoma was related.

The rheumatoid arthritis had started prior to his joining the service. He had not listed it on his application to join the army, fearing it would make him ineligible. Lacking other resources for school, hoping to qualify for college help through the GI bill, and mostly, wanting to help the country that had saved his Jewish mother from the Nazis, he was determined to be a soldier.

Once there, in Vietnam, he lost whatever faith he had in God or in the cause—the war—in which his country was engaged. But he, nonetheless, fulfilled his obligation, survived, was 100% service-connected, as we termed it in the VA medical system. He studied chemistry for some time in college, then trained as an auto-mechanic, doing this work until he was no long able to hold tools, the rheumatoid arthritis deforming his hands. I wondered if the auto-shop work had been the nidus of his WD-40 self-treatment...

"You look silver," I told him now. I didn't really have any other words for it, though "silver" wasn't a sign or symptom of anything with which I was familiar.

Again, that sparkly grin and "It's my silver flask, probably."

This was a little worrisome. Certainly, alcoholism had been present in many of my VA patients, especially those who had suffered trauma—which was pretty much all of them. In Mormon Utah, alcohol was often thought of as dangerous in any form or amount, but in residency, and in my work at the VA, we had learned to be appropriately concerned about problem-drinking, but accepting of social, occasional use, even understanding the possible health benefits of limited amounts of red wine. It was sometimes tricky though—quantifying. A patient once told me he had only one drink a day—which turned out to be a super-big-gulp cup—of hard liquor...

Fritz pulled out a blessedly small silver flask.

"What's in it?" I asked.

"My silver."

When he had used the words "silver flask" I was transported back to my own chemistry days, in high school, in fact. Our excellent, worn-out teacher, Mr. Hilton, who seemed to lack the energy to make unruly students work. When no one seemed to be paying attention as he wrote chemical equations on the board, or reviewed properties of elements, he would simply stop, slump-shrug, and say, "Well. Oh, well."

Then inevitably someone would ask him to get out his bed of nails—a large board with so many nails in it that one could walk on it without pain or harm. This he did, and we would walk on it. It was amazing each time.

Or we'd ask him for the TV. Not to watch something, it was a broken television I suppose, on a tall wheeled case. He would wheel it out and some brave soul would volunteer to take hold of his pliers or wrench, both metal. Then we would all hold hands in a circle and the person with the tool gingerly applied it to the metal knob—at which point we all felt a jolt—the strongest electrical shock experienced by the one directly connected to the machine. Even then, pre-medical school, I hoped that that person had a strong heart, not predisposed to arrythmia, was not an epileptic, did not have metal braces... that sort of thing.

Sometimes people asked to go to Topper's for doughnuts. Mr.

Hamilton never exactly gave permission, but would say, "They have excellent apple fritters." And assuming that there was one on his desk when the Topper's "field trip" ended, he seemed unlikely to discipline the absent students. My friend Margot, an artist with a car, and I once asked if we could go to the Eccles Art Center. Nothing was happening in class, no one was paying attention, we both had all the assignments done. Mr. Hamilton raised an eyebrow, nothing more. And we went to the art center in downtown Ogden, to see her Aunt Julie's excellent oil paintings.

But the silver flask. When we learned about the element, silver, Mr. Hamilton showed us how he could use melted silver to coat anything, then did so with a silver flask—the glass beaker sort of flask used in a laboratory. It was absolutely beautiful, for some reason I was very drawn to it—especially when he said

"Anyone who finishes the class with more than 100%, will earn the silver flask."

Air fairy in her infancy then—maybe more just a drive to excel, or a competitive streak—I had to do it. It meant that I had to get 100% on every exam, plus correctly answer the bonus questions, do all assignments on time, attend and correctly complete all lab sessions, and participate in class. And I did it. And earned the silver flask. I kept it for years, though now I don't know where it is, and still feel a little sad. I wonder if I could buy or make one. I really liked it.

But back to Felix.

"Silver? Why do you have a flask of silver? Silver inside—not just the flask?"

"Colloidal silver, Doc," he replied. "I started taking it a few weeks or a few months or—well honestly a year or so ago. I read that it would help cure my lymph, my cancer. Nothing else seems to be working."

I don't know exactly what to say. I start to say something about it being toxic, my fear that it might be damaging his organs, his kidneys, even his brain. His cancer treatment is done at the VA, so I am not always aware of the details of his regimens. But I know that the chemotherapy and radiation have not been successful in curing it, though possibly they have prolonged his life. And, at least between cycles of treatment, it has kept him going, able to get around, fight infection well enough to see friends, go to his coffee shop, feed the migratory birds at Liberty Park. And yet—his treatments have included clear poisons— and radiation. How much more harmful is his silver therapy?

I end up telling him this. He seems to appreciate the irony, the honesty. I get my laptop—still I resist technology in the room between me and my patient—and together, we look up "colloidal silver" on Google. We find a Mayo Clinic article that tells us about argyria, a condition of blue-grey—though in his case silver—tinting of the skin, eyes, organs, nails, gums, etc. that can occur with buildup of the silver in tissues over time. And it does cause kidney damage, can cause seizures, can interact with certain antibiotics and thyroid and other medicines. We decide to do lab work, checking his kidneys, thyroid, blood counts—and I do advise stopping the colloidal silver.

He gives me a sparkling grin. Silver gums, it's true. He asks for my pen. I hand it to him. He pours some silver on it, a few drops, it glows, it's pretty. He hands it back.

"Thanks, Felix," I say.

"Thanks, Doc." He re-masks and waits for my MA to come draw his blood, then schedules a follow-up for the next month.

I tell Dragon his story, careful to document my advice against using the silver. I wonder if I should have been more forceful in my condemnation of his use of the toxic compound. I wonder if the silver pen on my desk resembles an apple fritter.

My List

Were I to write an essay on hope now... well perhaps it would be but a poem. Or even merely a list. Of things I love, of reasons to work.

"Wake up," I command Dragon. I am going to tell him my list:

Old roses.

Rockstar's dark brown eyes; his white ruff, soft as heaven, the sounds he makes when he sleeps near.

April, my goddaughter, her corn-silk hair and her light brown eyes.

Her questions, her inventions.

Running fast.

Opening the lid of a grand piano, adjusting the bench, playing a note.

The blue-green oceans and endless headlands of Mendocino.

Llama eyelashes.

Fuchsia foxgloves near bright lime-green moss.

The sound of a river, a blackbird... of windchimes... of rain.

Heated blankets, poems spoken by heart, fairy stories, spiced tea.

Times when I'm warm and safe and harmless and grateful, known and still loved.

My Trade

For mind training, for beginners
the instruction is to start with something simple,
something you do every day: for example,
brushing your teeth:
notice mind, thoughts, breath, then return to the task

but this mind, and these thoughts!

That these teeth are the product of illness—
my own disease that left them weak,
broken;
my work, a physician, is the illness of others—
I mean, my trade—
to buy my teeth

Or this— each tooth in my mouth:
a small fortune,
the set in entirety would feed dozens, hundreds
(the five-thousand?)
hordes of starving people.

People for teeth. My trade.

Does a bright white smile gain me entry into the kingdom
of heaven
or hell?

Gritty mint, swish and spit,
Cool and burning,
Teeth burnished bright.

Return mind to breath, this mind, this priceless breath.

Two Major Surgeries and Two Major Marathons

I did not start running until well into my thirties, relatively recently, really, though having crossed forty, and with the strangeness of pandemic time, it seems long ago. I mean, I ran and was pretty fast as a little girl, and sometimes I tried to run until I couldn't breathe or couldn't make my legs go any longer—but that wasn't really a "long run," a term with which I quickly gained familiarity as I trained for a marathon. I am not sure why I started training, exactly. But the reason I continued? I loved it. I, me, Melissa, not Air Fairy. Being outside; having a bit of a community amongst runners, something a bit novel and lovely: being able to think, or to not think. And yet...Could there be an activity more perfect for her, Air Fairy, I mean, of course. Keep going, ignore body-mind weakness, blisters, shin splints, pouring rain, freezing snow, exhaustion, biting flies, brine flies (my first marathon was from Antelope Island in the Great Salt Lake into downtown Layton, UT). And yet I, me, not Air Fairy, loved running too. So, maybe Air Fairy is part of me, or impossibly intertwined, despite Dr. Hardy's best efforts at separation, exorcism. I'm not masochistic, I don't like feeling pain. I do like feeling tougher = safer = stronger. I do like feeling fast and... and I don't know—is it a sport, an art, a hobby? Where is it harmful, a new way of training, not in running, but in denial of bodily needs or discomforts?

I started running with a friend, Chavez, who has a doctorate in physical therapy and owns a physical therapy clinic to which I often refer patients. I think he is an amazing runner and a good friend. He made me run "the toll road" a seemingly endless, impossibly-steep climb from the mouth of Weber Canyon up a road bridge, passing over train tracks, river, through toll booths (no charge for runners—the cost is just the laughter of the attendants as you try not to throw up, face beet-red, try not to pass out). Then, finally, cresting at the far southeast end of the hospital grounds, at which point I would want to collapse, but be coaxed to "walk it out." Too tired to argue, I walked, with Chavez patting me on the back and telling me how he took the new orthopedic PA "up the toll road last week. He puked his guts. Good job." Is it horrible that I felt a bit proud?

"When we were young on the farm in Blackfoot," he would say, "we used to carry the littlest kids on our backs while we picked corn or dug potatoes, onions. Then we ran with 50-pound bags of potatoes in our arms and 50-pound kids on our backs."

"You ran with them?" I would ask. "Why?"

"To save time and the kids had fun."

"Oh. Wow."

"We did it without shoes. In the snow, middle of winter."

"Oh. Wow. Wait. Why were you harvesting fields in the middle of winter, how does that make sense?"

He did not seem to hear me.

But he also told me to eat. More. Food. And that I was a good runner but would be better, could be better, should weigh more if I wanted to be better. So, Dr. Hardy likes him, his wanting me to be larger, be fed, eat food, not air. Chavez and I have lost touch a bit, he had meniscus surgery I had—well, two major surgeries (read on)… and then there was that pandemic...

"What did Chavez say you should weigh to run?" Dr. Hardy will ask.

"It wasn't that, it was not a specific instruction, training advice with evidence behind it—it was just a throw-away comment of his, maybe," I say.

"You are throwing away the friendship of a kind, hard-working man, who tries to help you achieve your goals?" he said.

"No, that's not what I meant, or said, I mean... We just haven't seen each other, the pandemic, I said it was a throw-away comment, not throwing away friendship..."

Other than with Chavez, I ran alone. Oh, heavens, not alone, with Rockstar, my pup. But I confess, I did enjoy running with someone. Talking, or, since usually I was out of breath, listening. At some point, I must have mentioned it to my dad that I was running, and running with someone. My dad loves being a grandpa, perhaps more than anything.

"Him?" my dad said. "The person you are running with is male?"

"Um. Yes."

"A male human person? Not a patient, you are running together for fun?"

"Yes, Dad, or, well, for training, sort of, to try to be a better runner, for me. But, Dad, he is 25 years older and—."

"That's okay, that's fine, not much difference."

"—and he is happily married with children and—"

"Oh. Okay."

But. Chavez was supremely tough. In addition to work, unofficial training with referring clinicians, time with his wife and kids, he spent time teaching troubled young men how to box. Chavez had boxed with Joe Frazier, "fought against Ali's guys." He, Chavez, was an alternate U.S. Olympic Team boxer. And he had a 2:15 marathon. I did not (of course), but we ran the Huntsville marathon together—mostly together, though not talking, and he finished a few minutes ahead: we rode up together on the bus, strategized about stashing Honey Stinger Waffles in bra (me) or forearm strap bag (him). We saw a moose along the run. And I finished at 3:20, not any record of course, but 3rd woman overall, even though I was oldish. And I got a trophy. It was a bit big, and totally wonderful.

And it was a fast enough time to qualify for Boston. Which I decided to do. And did. I ran the Boston Marathon the following year, with a disappointingly slow 4:04:52 time. Here is why.

It is typical for sage runners to advise negative splits—or just not starting out too fast, pacing. An observer looking at a mile-by-mile record of my pace during that Boston run might have guessed that that was the problem, starting out too fast, being forced to slow down with fatigue as the miles wore on. As the one running, the body running, I know that the problem was that my intestines fell out at mile eight. That beautiful morning, surrounded by breathtaking masses of Bostoners, out to support anonymous runners sprinting or struggling through their city. I was listening to them cheer us on, feeling the pavement and the vibration of hundreds or thousands of feet hitting it along with mine… and then feeling the awful internal intestinal drop.

They didn't all fall out, of course, and it wasn't the first time. I have a progressive chronic illness characterized by loss of supportive tissues. This includes the mesentery and fat pads that hold the abdominal organs and intestines in place. It is something to which I gave little thought, how vital organs remain in place in a body, a seldom-celebrated marvelous bit of anatomy: tissues of incredible strength, flexibility, and softness, fat and sinew, cradle, encasement.

But in me, they started to fail, to disintegrate, to be consumed. Then, things do fall apart.

So, the intestines falling out didn't happen all at once, and Boston was not the first time. In retrospect, subtle rectal prolapse began for me in high school, though I didn't know what it was. I did at one point mention it to my trusted and kind family medicine doctor, who did not, however, do an exam. He assumed it was hemorrhoids and then neither of us really mentioned it again, no treatment or assessment. So it seemed to me, or Air Fairy, not a problem, unless I made it one. And I was tough, or could be, or should be. I could push things back in. They would sag out over the course of a day, especially if standing or walking or running—but then that is just another chance to be tougher, not a reason to sit. Unfortunately, things started to come apart in a way that led to the intestines being kinked, obstructed at times—and that was painful, tough for Air Fairy even.

When running, often, some amount of prolapse would occur, and, well, I would just run a bit bowlegged, I guess. And it was not predictable and didn't always happen. Sometimes it seemed if I didn't eat it wouldn't happen, maybe nothing in the intestines. It seems plausible then they would be lighter and stay inside. But it is tough to run a marathon without eating for days before. Tough even for Air Fairy. So, Boston. Was bad. I ran and then would try to inconspicuously push things back up through the rectum, squeeze together, hold everything in, and still run. I waddled, I fear. There is a picture, one that the race drones or cameramen take along the way. My face is "a mask of pain" as they say. And my stance says it all, knees bent, thighs strangely apart, taut exhaustion.

So. I might have mentioned it to my mother, who had come with me and met me after the rally, as a reason I was not very fast or why I slowed pace at mile eight. And I did not want to walk very far to the car, then the airport, the gate. Sitting on the plane, a mix of pride at having finished anyway, humiliation at slowness, and slight, perpetually squashed horror at my body falling apart. I loved running. How could I run and eat and hold together?

Eventually my gastroenterologist had me see a colorectal surgeon, Dr. Mindy Blackwell. Who, for the first time in the 20 years this had been happening, did an examination. And then did a series of horrific tests including essentially having a barium bowel movement on a radiology toilet with radiopaque objects in my rectum and vagina while being watched and recorded by the radiologist.

Dr. Blackwell: "You need surgery, but I won't do it."

Me: "Oh."

Dr. Blackwell: "The surgery is an open abdominal procedure, with removal of problematic bowel and reanastamosis, reattaching. I am the best person to do it."

Me: "Oh, um, that's great."

Dr. Blackwell: "So, if you want to have it done you have to weigh 100 pounds or more. Otherwise, it is too risky. You may not heal and be left with an ostomy, no working intestines."

Me: "Oh."

Dr. Blackwell: "So we will place a PICC line and start TPN, here is a card with the information, but stop at the desk around the corner and Jeana will get things scheduled."

Me: "But…" But she has gone.

But, I work full time as an internist, seeing patients, how exactly am I to have an open abdominal surgery, where is there time for that? But, TPN is horrific, when I was a resident and hospitalist we learned never to use it. It stands for Total Parenteral Nutrition, essentially food given in an IV. But, it leads to complete failure of the GI system, if nothing is going into the stomach, bowels, they stop working entirely. Now, we also would worry about effects on microbiome, the millions of bacteria inhabiting the GI tract, whose functions include immunity, hormone regulation, metabolism, much more. On the other hand, other pathogenic bacteria, as well as sometimes deadly fungi, have a perfect pathway to the blood with TPN USE— they feed on the nutrients in the line, leading to bloodstream infection. That is, pathogens had easy access through the PICC, short for Peripherally Inserted Central Catheter—perhaps from a contaminated nurse's glove—introducing them into the central veins, right along with the nutritive solution, the TPN. Overwhelming sepsis could occur with horrific speed. And, how exactly was I to do this anyway, while seeing patients and...

But, I did it. With intestines not staying in place, I couldn't eat and also stand, and work, not enough to gain the weight Dr. Blackwell stipulated was necessary to decrease the risks of her planned surgery. So, I did the TPN. Until my weight with jeans and winter boots was enough, just before the end of the year. The timing was in some ways fortunate—I had met my out-of-pocket insurance maximum, and I could try to schedule a few extra days off around the holidays, when things were maybe slower, or at least the clinic was closed for the holidays.

The surgery was late in the evening. Though my parents had been there, afterwards, they left. It must have been quite late by then, they must have wanted to get home to bed. I vaguely remember them there—in the interval between coming out of the post-op area and falling asleep again. It had apparently gone well, been successful, but went several hours long. When I awoke in the night, the first time I was really awake after anesthesia, I got up to go to the bathroom—and collapsed. There was surely a call button for the nurse, somewhere, but I knew nurses are all overstretched, covering too many patients, and, surely I could go to the bathroom myself, it was steps from my bed. But I had, after all, been disemboweled, I suppose: a cut across my low abdomen. The pain pump, which was supposed to deliver on-demand narcotic at the push of a button, was not connected, not set up, so my desperate, reaching, pressing thumb was ineffective.

I was incontinent then. And on the floor and freezing cold, mostly naked. After a bit, a nurse came in, and indeed she did appear overstretched and tired, and seemed most displeased with the mess I made—myself, my fluids, the bed linens all on the floor.

An Air Fairy failure. I cried a bit. But over the next days I walked endlessly and did not take pain medicine and got out of the hospital as quickly as I could. I was to continue the TPN, the idea being maximal nutrition for healing and allowing things to hold together inside without excessive food weight, meaning weight in the intestines. Letting them rest. However, on New Year's Eve I experienced rigors, uncontrollable shaking chills, in the middle of the night. This was a condition about which I had read in textbooks, maybe seen once or twice, but never experienced. And really I had no concept. I. Could. Not. Get. Warm. Or stop shaking. Somehow, after some time, I got my cell phone and, ridiculously, made a video, knowing I would not be able to describe what was happening to doctors, not knowing how to make them realize it was a problem. I tried to reach the on-call surgeon.

Eventually, I went to the ER of my hospital, the hospital where I worked at the time, as a hospitalist. It was just across the street from the condo where I lived. They pulled the PICC line, drew labs, and confirmed bacteremia. They also noted liver compromise, but, ultimately, after an antibiotic injection, and with the line out, I stopped shaking. Fortunately, the ER doctor was a sympathetic colleague—and knew that I lived just across the street so if anything got worse, I could come back—they let me go home. They are always busy New

Year's Eve anyway; it would have been hard to want to talk another patient into staying.

Sometime the next day the on-call surgeon called me back and said it was good the line was pulled, or something like that, and to take antibiotics. I, foolishly, or bravely, or trying to reassert my toughness, or determined to start the new year out well—went to the Antelope Island First Day hike with my pup. Air Fairy success. PICC line and TPN gone. Intestines inside body again. Get on with things, life, work...

*   *   *

I loved the New York City marathon. I ran it in 2019, the last time it was held before the pandemic. I was struggling to be anywhere near my previous speed, but I was in. Running across the bridge, through the five boroughs was amazing. And amazingly hard. My intestines stayed in, though their contents were liquid and churning most of the time. But that is normal. "Runner's diarrhea." Wimpy to think about. I was glad to be there, running into Central Park where my dad was waiting. And the weather was cool, there was the slightest rain. There were masses of people, but there was an unusual—in my limited New York experience—spirit of camaraderie and even celebration. My dad got a taxi. I was glad to finish. I was not fast.

Around that time, I started having strange headaches. And losing my sense of position and my ability to stay upright. I fell down my stairs. My home—where I live now, having left the condo for the capital city and my small downtown clinic—was built in 1927. It is absolutely beautiful, in a national and local historic district. Tudor, I think. Well-made. Beautiful, steep, narrow wooden stairs. Cherry wood trim—it made me think, inexplicably, of a small sailing ship—maybe something about the wood and small neat perfectly designed cupboards and railings. The polished steps glowed. And I completely fell down all of sixteen of them.

But. Headaches. Dizziness. Really? How often is that a complaint? As an internist I will tell you: very often. And nothing is wrong. Only wimpiness. But the stairs... did worry me. With osteoporotic bones…that could make it hard to walk, let alone run. Or to work.

By then I had an established internist looking after me, someone who had helped train me, in residency. When I finally told him of the headaches—back of head and neck, occurring with pressure, such as sneezing/coughing/bowel movement—he did ask about family history. And on learning that my little brother had a cerebral AVM that bled—he ordered a brain scan. Which showed that my brain was falling out.

There is something called a chiari malformation, which describes herniation of the cerebellum into the cervical spine—a part of the brain a bit lower in the skull, so that it is at the top of the neck. If there is 5mm of herniation, that is considered significant, a consideration for surgery if the person with it has headaches or other symptoms. My cerebellum and brain stem herniated 28mm and were compressed, stuck down in the cervical spinal canal. A chiari malformation in general is thought to be congenital. In my case, it seemed, the supportive tissue around the brain, the fat pad at the base of the skull, the tissues to keep everything in the skull that should be, rather than sliding down into the spine—was gone. So brain falling...

I met with a neurologist, who showed the film to a neurosurgeon. At which time, I was interrupted in afternoon clinic with a phone call. Which I did not want to take, but was told it was another doctor needing to speak with me.

Me: "Hello?"

Person on the phone: "Hi, Melissa, this is Andrea from Dr. Schmidt's office, we need you to come in."

Me: "Dr. Schmidt?"

Andrea: "Yes, Robert Schmidt, can you come now? We are at the main neurosciences building—"

Me, interrupting: "No, I'm in the middle of clinic. I have next Friday off if he has a time then."

Andrea: "Um, you need to come now I think."

Ultimately, I went. Seeing me I think was reassuring for the good neurosurgeon, Dr. Schmidt. He said I needed surgery. But I seemed intact. Intact. Great.

"There is a pandemic, only emergent surgeries are being done now," I said.

"Yep," he said. "I am ordering dexamethasone for you to take for the next day or two until we operate, and we'll get you in a c-collar, I am not sure if we have one small enough…" he was heading for the door.

So it seemed I was an emergency.

"But," I said. This time loudly, and not letting him leave the room. "I am not having brain surgery."

He said nothing.

"My little brother had brain surgery. He is fine, but not really. I am a doctor. It is the only thing I do that matters. Even if the surgery goes well, from your standpoint, from almost any standpoint, if anything is at all off, I can't be a doctor, I will do harm, it will not be okay, I will not be okay. I am fine. I can manage headaches, they are fine. I can take Tylenol. I can do PT (physical therapy) so that I don't fall anymore, I can work on balance."

To summarize: I got another opinion from Mayo, thank the pandemic for virtual consult options. They agreed to have me come there for assessment, and agreed that I seemed, yes, intact. But they had me do a sleep study, which showed severe central sleep apnea. Not the more common obstructive sleep apnea in which, sometimes due to large body habitus, or just bad anatomy or genetic luck, the airway closes off at night blocking the airway transiently. Central sleep apnea is caused by a brain problem. For example, the brain stem, with respiratory centers in the medulla oblongata, getting squished against cervical vertebrae.

And, I developed episodic hand numbness. Sometimes it seemed random, though it predictably happened if I tipped my head back. And the neurosurgeon said that I might develop irreversible upper extremity weakness. Difficult to be a doctor—let alone play the piano, paint, draw, manage an Australian shepherd on-leash sighting squirrels on neighborhood walks—without well-working hands.

Me: "What are the risks?"

Dr. Graystone, the Mayo neurosurgeon: "Of having surgery? Just to be clear."

This was progress. That I was even considering it.

Me: "Yes."

Dr. Graystone: "It's possible that it won't help, or that you will have a different type of headache. In my time at Rochester, I saw a patient who had her vertebral artery severed and had a devastating stroke."

Me: "That's bad."

Dr. Graystone: "In my hands, there is almost no chance of an adverse event. I consider it an adverse event if the surgery doesn't resolve symptoms, dramatically improve your headaches and balance. And that doesn't happen, in my hands."

And so, I put myself into the perfect hands of the Dr. Graystone for surgery, at the Mayo Clinic in Arizona.

He came to see me before I was wheeled in. I was alone, staying at a hotel on the hospital campus, which was convenient. And I didn't need anyone there. Really. I had a rental car, but had walked across the parking lot for surgery. They told me to leave my wallet, money anything else with family—or in any case not to bring it to the hospital. So I didn't bring anything. I took off my clothes and put on the gown and answered the anesthesia pre-op questions.

When Dr. Graystone came in to see me before the operation it was around noon, and they were close to start time.

"Hello, Dr. Bentley," he said.

"Hi, Dr. Graystone," I said.

"Whom should I call when we are done?" he asked.

"Umm," I said. My father had decided he only wanted to be a grandpa, was giving up on children, too worrisome and no way to help and not very life-affirming. And he didn't like to hear about or talk about anything sad or scary or negative. My mother and stepfather were living in Europe.

"You are alone here, staying at the Marriott on the hospital campus, is that right?" he confirmed. He had told me this was okay. We planned accordingly that, although hard to predict, I would likely be in the hospital for about five days. Usual stay was three days for this surgery, with him—and he anticipated mine might be a bit complicated. So, the additional days in hospital might help with nutrition and rest afterwards, rather than leaving me to my own care (or Air Fairy's).

"Yes," I said.

After checking with Dr. Hardy to be sure it was okay, I gave the surgeon my psychologist's, Dr. Hardy's, phone number.

And I remember nothing of the surgery, itself, of course. I was cold and then I was warm and then I was asleep.

The following day, I couldn't stop sleeping. At some point the neurosurgery fellow came by. Hours passed. I knew I should get up, be awake, and I couldn't. Apparently, the nurse told me, I only had fentanyl available for pain, and she had been giving it to me. I must have asked her to stop it, because then I had pain. My skull had been cut open, a piece of bone removed. Another piece of bone was removed from my cervical vertebrae. They had planned to use pericranial tissue to create a type of cushion or mesh, but there wasn't any tissue. So they used titanium mesh. I suppose that cutting into bone would explain pain. I asked for Tylenol, which was also something I had orders for. And then I asked for it again—but my orders were for 325mg tablets, 2 of them every 8 hours if needed. It had not been eight hours; so I could have fentanyl and be asleep again or have unbearable pain, until they could reach a prescriber.

I did not see Dr. Graystone. A physical therapist supposedly came by. There is a law that enables patients to view their records, which I have since done. There are notes that indicate the PT was told I was up and around and didn't need him. Which is not true. I struggled to find my phone or laptop. Rather, I knew they were in a bag on a chair, located an impossible four feet from my bed. I could not stand or stay awake. I needed to notify people or see if there was a message or…

Eventually I saw the nurse and asked if it was okay to eat. She said, "Of course, go ahead."

And left before I could ask how or what to eat.

And the next time I saw her she informed me, "They have discharged you, so you are free to go."

I was stunned.

And had to try to stay awake.

"Um… I still have a catheter and I haven't eaten anything or stood up or…"

"Oh, let's get the catheter out, we have this new method called fill-and-pull, so I'll go get the supplies…" and she left.

And I could not stay awake.

I was discharged. I managed to have them wait until I had been told how to order food and ordered a boiled egg and I did not take anything for pain so that I kept myself awake, and had pain.

I had a bite of egg.

Fortunately, the discharge aide put me in a wheelchair and took me to the discharge pharmacy. They had ordered oxycodone, which I was very reluctant to get, everything worrisome about opiates from my experience as a doctor and what I had read and seen—but also my head really hurt and I had no idea how I was going to sleep, no part of it didn't hurt—how would I lie on a pillow?

I also had no wallet, having been advised to leave it outside. With insurance, my cost was thirty-four cents, which the aide graciously offered to pay. I thanked her but found a $20 bill I'd stashed in my backpack.

She got me a water bottle and got me onto the shuttle to the hotel. I couldn't stand up. The shuttle driver helped me get my wallet from my car to re-check in at my hotel. I had not been able to change the reservation that was made for a few days hence, since I was told to plan on five days. But when told I was being discharged, I couldn't find a number or phone or stay awake long enough to do so from the hospital.

The front desk woman, "Name?"

"Bentley, Melissa. I had a reservation for later this week but am discharged and…"

"Hmm. Let me see what I can do…"

While she was seeing what she could do, I was falling over and collapsed into a lobby chair.

"Sorry, just need to sit."

I was not sure she heard me above her tapping fingernails. But she found a room and somehow I got into it and into, or at least on top of the bed. I took an oxycodone and fell asleep.

It was the only time I took the oxycodone, as it caused terrible nausea, and I could not vomit or my skull would fall apart, I feared. When I was able to communicate with Dr. Hardy, and read the operative report, I learned it had been an eight-hour procedure. That there had not been any pericranial tissue, so they used titanium to create a supportive mesh. Neither of us had any idea why I was discharged.

Or, that isn't exactly true. I could guess. Once upon a time, as a resident, I did surgery rotations, I remember having a service of five, ten, fifteen patients, more coming in for admission post-surgery, trying to get to all of them on pre-rounds. Then get orders in, check the orders, review results, change the orders. I remember the drive to discharge, to "diurese" the service, both simply to physically be able to manage the patients for whom I was responsible, and to make room. Frequently hospitals had reminders to discharge by noon, even had whole "discharge teams" at times, with sole purpose of going through the hospital floors, checking with the primary teams, and writing orders for discharge for any patient felt stable enough to go. Then too, understandably, with the COVID pandemic, there were no spare resources: nurses, doctors, beds, masks, ventilators, time, and care were all scarce and precious.

I spent days walking the thankfully level trails around the hospital, the hotel, looking at birds, cacti, though without moving my head. No looking up, cautious turning side-to-side. I found the very best cold pack, it was Snoopy, the Peanuts character, at a local CVS store. I tried in vain in the weeks ahead to find another, calling stores, writing, checking online—it was exactly the right size and combination of firmness and softness—I wanted another to keep one always frozen. I loved it and still have it today. With that and lots of Tylenol—children's Tylenol, since the adult capsules or tablets hurt my pitifully wimpy previously damaged stomach or intestines—I managed. I had arm swelling and really awful face swelling, and an impressive wound from the crown of my head to the middle of my upper back.

Maybe the hardest thing—or one of the hardest things—is that I did not feel at all well, and I had admitted it—I told the nurse and, when I saw him, even in my half-asleep fentanyl state—I told the neurosurgery fellow that I was not well enough. I was not ready for discharge, I couldn't stand up or stay awake, I had not eaten. And it didn't matter. And all of that was just weakness anyway.

Air Fairy knew it. I had not paid attention to her, had failed, and clearly it was wrong. I was fine. I didn't die, was discharged and fine. And there was a pandemic. People everywhere were dying. I was using resources that should have been used elsewhere, I was focused on myself, forgetting the larger world and the very real need for care for the thousands of COVID patients who became sick and often died, daily. The health care system, the people in it providing the care, were stretched beyond capacity. Beyond the capacity to care or translate the emotional caring into physical care of the sick.

So. Eventually I went home and—an eternity or mandatory six weeks later—I went back to work. And—Air Fairy, please be quiet—it was a bit hard. My clinic got me a different computer desk with two larger screens, adjustable height, and with time it was possible to keep neck and head in check and… and I love being a doctor and was, am, so glad to be at work. As a doctor. Done being the patient. Sort of.

Now, as I finish writing this essay, I am not really running yet, not allowed to, though I am registered for the Chicago Marathon this fall, having twice deferred through pandemic years. I do run at the Crimson Lagoon, the beautiful aquatic complex at the University of Utah. I wear a flotation belt and run long laps in the cold pool, or, on wimpy days, I wear water-running shoes and run in the warmer activity pool; often a combination of the two. I go very early, and some days it is just me and a lifeguard. I love the idea of someone guarding my life—from what, or whom? How? Of course, so I don't drown…

I am hoping that another major marathon, if I manage it someday, post-pandemic, does not mean another major surgery. It is hard to look far ahead. It is hard to see the back of my head, after surgery, to check for any sign of wound dehiscence or infection. I could do it using my cell phone camera, after lots of tries and photos of my shirt or collar or the space above my head. Or using multiple opposing mirrors. Better to not look at the wounded part, to be tough.

From the front no one would know I had brain surgery. And my intestines are all inside my body.

My body buttoned up in its white coat.

Animal Interlude

Animals—mostly foxes and owls; and, of course, a dog, my Australian shepherd, Rockstar, features a bit. But not much of Air Fairy or Dragon. Though my work is, maybe, the only thing I do that matters. The only thing I can do in a unique and possibly useful way—on a good day, with fullest concentration of my efforts and with God's grace.

In any case, this interlude is a chance to breathe. No medical practice in this chapter, I don't think. It seeps in sometimes, being a doctor—it saturates, matters so much to me, that it likely does color the way I see and experience and understand the world. But no Dragon here and only the bits of Air Fairy that, after 40 years, I fear are also subtly and solidly incorporated into my being. Are they me or—I guess I mean—am I them?

First, owls. I took a class at the local botanical garden, Red Butte Gardens, called "Owl Portraits." I loved it. The instructor, Elaine, was a wonderful artist. She was also often very vague, distracted-seeming, scattered or unfocused to the point of also being oblivious. It may have been just her creativity or artistic nature—and I may be sorely lacking in that realm—but at times, at first, being with her could make me feel a bit desperate, frustrated. Why are we not moving on, where are instructions, why is she wandering around sort of looking at what students are doing, but not really in a systematic way, and then stopping, and then having us all come to the front to watch—what? She seemed to forget by the time she was back to where she started.

"Does anyone see my lemon yellow penc—never mind, it is here, okay. Good. Fine. Can you all see?" she said, as we surrounded her.

"Oh, Elaine, look at that, the color you achieved for the orchid petals, what was your base layer?" a student asked, and then it was ages, it seemed, before we were back to our—well, to the drawing technique she was detailing, I thought.

"I make sure it is sharp, the pencil, create a sweet spot," Elaine began.

"Is that paper the Strathmore?" another student, Julie, asked. I fear I sighed then, wanting to get on with it, learn, watch, then go do my drawing...

"No, Julie, do you all have—in your folders, there should be a small manila envelope with paper samples, do you all have that?" Elaine asked.

"Yes, thank you," I said quickly, "I am sure we all have that. Ready for your demonstration of—something important." But. Off we were sent, back to our desks to check our registration packets to be sure the paper swatches had indeed been included. Then back to surround Elaine to see how to properly use mechanical or electric pencil sharpeners and then…

Then we learned about owls. Using an overhead projector—honestly, they still exist. The type with clear films on which a teacher can write with marker, images showing on a white pull-down screen. Projections of whole owls and wings, single feathers and talons. And their faces. Individual faces that each looked like an individual, even if the same species. We learned which owl species are found in Utah (there are probably fourteen!). Where they nest, ground or trees—where to go in the Salt Lake region to see them. It was nature, or biology, or art—but it was magical. In moments, for moments, I just looked and drew. I would say or write that I enjoyed it, but it isn't that, quite. I just—well I just wasn't. *I* wasn't. No Melissa, no Dr. Bentley, no pandemic, patients, not anything—only just colored pencils and paper and shapes and lines. Looking and learning, listening.

I needed a grayed-lavender Prismacolor pencil, which for some reason seemed to be a hot item in town. I had not found it at the local Blick, in Sugarhouse, when I was getting the supply list items specified in the Class Welcome email. I had to make a second trip and get suggestions for other possible shops. This was my problem? It sort of made me laugh, definitely smile. Could there be a more lovely dilemma than struggling to find a grayed-lavender pencil? No one would die or become infected with a deadly virus if I didn't find it.

I knew nothing about drawing with colored pencils, really. I could make a complete mess of the whole affair, fail to find the right supplies, draw an owl that looks like a bat or a ghost. Even make a literal mess—pencil sharpening shavings on the carpet, extraneous scraps of paper strewn about—no one minded. If anything, they anticipated it—it was expected, there was surprise when I asked where the waste and recycling bins were. The Garden volunteers would clean up the classroom later. Don't worry about it. Just enjoy your time with Elaine.

It was similar, but completely different too—to the way it feels when I slip into my white coat. I disappeared—no self in view, in the way. Just the patient, the illness or dilemma. Or, in this case, the colors, hook of beak, texture of feathers, pressure of pencil, grain of paper.

For a field trip, we had planned to go to the Tracy Aviary—which has owls. Unfortunately, there was a blizzard, an April snowstorm. Gale-force wind, then nickel or quarter sized snowflakes, inches of heavy snow on the ground almost instantly. The field trip was canceled, or, more hopefully, postponed. But this is, in fact, a weather phenomenon not so unusual in Utah. And the birds are still there, they still receive care at the almost-always-open Aviary. And (minor Air Fairy sighting), snow did not interrupt my planned runs. Too wimpy, not allowed. So, I ran at Liberty Park. This park encompasses the Aviary, as well as a huge pond, a run-down amusement park, a homeless encampment.

The next part of this story seems impossible. But, it happened. I think. Again, it seems another person's life, another lifetime. But. Here it is. I had a boyfriend. At the time, Andy. And there is much to write about that, but I am not going to, at least not now. What I want to describe is this. I ran around the park. The outer trail is a 1.5 mile circle, and I was doing 12 miles—eight times around. After I had done maybe three, I saw Andy, driving his black BMW, circling the roads near the pedestrian path. He was looking for me.

I watched as he drove slowly along, his car practically the only one on the streets. In it, he was inching around the park perimeter, making sure I was okay. Then he saw me and got out. He held up a Hudson Bay blanket into which he collected me as I shivered through the final steps of my last lap. He spread the blanket the way that a mother holds out a towel for her child emerging from a bath, or from the pool after a swim. Then, Andy bundled me into his warm car and we drove to the Aviary entrance, where we paid for tickets. I suspect we were the only visitors that day. I saw no one else, other than the employees.

We found owls. Since my hands were too frozen to use and he didn't want to get his cell phone/camera wet, we took no owl pictures—I had planned to use them for drawing. Instead, we just watched. My mouth, whole face were also numb, even in my balaclava/ski mask—which covering also made it hard for me to hear much. We just were silent with owls. Maybe in awe.

And there were many problems, with Andy, and with me of course, and the world. But the thing is, there was still that—that moment. Or those moments. Looking for grayed-lavender, and owls; being found and hugged into a blanket.

I met Andy before I met Rockstar. Before I met Rockstar, I considered dog ownership carefully. For probably 18 months. Serious consideration, I mean, not just "Oh, it might be nice to have a dog." Dr. Hardy helped me, of course.

"I don't think I—I am afraid I would be harmful for a dog," I said.

"Why?" he asked.

"Well, I have—I would want to do a good job, and I work and…"

"And Air Fairy takes a lot of time and attention, and maybe you would rather tend to her than…" he started.

"No," I interrupted. "It's just—it's just I have to be able to work and I just—I don't know. If things are dirty or not sorted then I might lose focus and then make a mistake or…"

He has three lovely dogs. Had then and has again. They are beautiful and smart, well-trained.

One day, Dr. Hardy saw the runt of a litter of Aussies on Facebook—he was on the social media site and I wasn't. There was a last pup, this runt, from a very good breeder in Payson, Utah, a small town about 2 hours south of Salt Lake City. He was at a kennel called Full Throttle's Australian Shepherds.

The puppy was adorable. Of course. I know all puppies are, but he was gorgeous and darling, both. I arranged to just go visit. To meet him. And then—I loved him. I think. I am always hesitant to write that I love someone or something—many times, I have read that it is not possible to love others if one doesn't love oneself. And—I think that is hard. Air Fairy doesn't need love and reminds me there is nothing about me that is lovable, and not to even think that is the case: that softness—arrogance. Selfish, self-centered, arrogant to think. Loving someone, or thinking someone loved me, inevitably might lead me to harm that person, somehow. Or to have an expectation of help if I needed it. And needing, desiring, is harmful. Plus, my work is to be a doctor. I do feel that I love my patients, but am aware it is a formal, structured love. Which doesn't mean it is easy or without peril.

In any case. I had to make a trip to Arizona for a work conference, which gave me a bit of time to think about dog ownership. Of this dog, in particular. And I wanted to try. The breeder, Liz at Full Throttle, was willing to take him back—in fact that was a condition of my buying him, the purchase contract. If it didn't work out, I would give him back. We were to be co-owners, Liz and I, until the dog was neutered.

So, when I got back, dear Andy drove with me to Payson. This was so that I could hold the pup—later to be officially named Rockstar—Full Throttle's Rocky Mountain Rockstar—while Andy drove me—or us—home.

It seems hard to believe, impossible, but Dr. Hardy helped me be a person who could—well, who could be a person for a dog. And not just any dog, but an Aussie. I took him with me to work, from the start. I had not asked permission exactly. I just did it. I took lessons on how to have a puppy from a wonderful woman named Nellie, who was also my patient. She had raised canine champions. And she loved doing dog hair, "big hair" was her thing. Nellie taught us door behavior, greeting behavior, "leave—it," the importance of a strong recall, the usefulness of pottying on command. The privilege of being a person for a dog. She helped us get our first "titles": Canine Good Citizenship, then Beginner Novice Obedience.

Rockstar. A name I chose because of the Rocky Mountains I love, where I live. And his rock-or-movie star eyelashes and self-assurance, swagger. And his Rockstar-drink level of energy and—who knows. It seemed cool, his name, his self—and I am decidedly uncool. But I suspected he would be called—and his call name for trials was—Rocky. So, driving back from Payson, I asked Andy to tell me about the Rocky movies—in case people thought that was why I named him that. Or in any case to be sure that Rocky—the person in the movie—was fine—that it wouldn't be a bad thing for Rocky the dog to be associated with him, Rocky Balboa of the films. There are so many Rocky films. Andy took me through each one. It was a long drive, so there was plenty of time. He seemed okay, Rocky Balboa, the movie star. Though, I confess my attention drifted at times, smitten by the adorable furball on my lap.

In any case. That is Rockstar, you know, from the title. And he will be featured plenty in this book. Maybe he is the star, truly, or my star, as corny as that sounds. My light.

A brief bit more about owls. They are hard to find, for me, in the wild. I took another owl art class, this one through continuing education at the university, and with watercolor as the medium. The class was in partnership with Hawkwatch International, an organization that rescues and provides healing space for injured birds. We had an owl from them, Sooki, as our model. Or Kooki. Or something. We were masked then, and I never quite caught his name from the soft-spoken artist-teacher, Natalya. The owl's longer full name was something like Kookatura—that is not right.

But he was beautiful. He would puff out his feathers suddenly, hack up an owl pellet, turn his head completely around, it seemed. This was also not long after pieces of my skull and cervical vertebrae had been removed, and I so envied that neck rotation! For me looking to the side—if I forgot for a moment that I'd had surgery and turned my head rather than just shifting my eyes, I was quickly reminded—by pain. Natalya was wonderful with watercolor, such fine delicate work. We were trying to do each feather, figure out how to give the idea of the bird's movement and presence. Natalya also knew and revealed to me where I could find great horned owls. They nested near the northwest edge of the Great Salt Lake. She told me exactly where they were and drew me a map.

It still took several tries, and binoculars, but I found them. Two. They were much larger than I expected. And so much like they are supposed to look, or like they do look, in pictures. Or in our classroom—but to see them sitting up in a tree, that silhouette was unmistakable. I could have stared a long time, mutual staring with the owls— even with my sore neck. But Rockstar spotted deer, and it was all I could do to keep him from plunging across the marsh after them.

I had also heard there was an owl at a near place, in my neighborhood, called Wasatch Hollow. During the pandemic, going to look for an owl was the perfect evening activity for Rockstar and me. It was hard, though, and the post-surgery pain from tipping my head back continued. Sometimes after a while looking up into the trees, my hands tingled or were numb, even when it wasn't cold out.

Then one day, Dr. Hardy told me of a fox. He had seen her in the old golf course, Bonneville Hills, near where we both live. We live a mile or so apart, on the foothills East of Salt Lake City. Proximity to Dr. Hardy was definitely a benefit of my chosen home location. Though not really an appropriate point to consider when relocating—boundary issues, yes?

In session:

"I did not see her. Still," I said.

"That is because you have to be slow and go in the middle of the afternoon. Be slow. On Sundays perhaps," he said. "You go for walks at six in the morning. It is dark and cold. Also, you walk too quickly, never stopping. She suns herself, this fox. You have to be more like a fox sunning herself on a patch of grass or a warm rock."

"Oh, okay," I said.

"Or not," he said. "Up to you."

I did not like it when he said that, for some reason.

"I want to see her," I said. And I did.

One winter day, scanning the snow-covered golf course, searching through trees, trying not to look too closely, as that seemed bad luck. If I admitted to myself or the world that I was desperately searching, I'd never see her. If I was nonchalant, simply out for a walk with my pup, then just maybe. But I did want to see her. I'd been searching for movement, the slight shift of a branch, and listening for a rustling of leaves, a crunch in the snow. Instead, I came upon her sleeping. She was like a tiny pool of tomato soup held in a porcelain snow cup. I fear I use the word "beautiful" too much—but she was. Just stunning, that orange-red, wrapped perfectly into herself, her head and ears and limbs all folded together, encircled by her thick tail. And, yes, she was indeed resting in a shaft of winter sun. It seemed—she seemed—so quiet. I am sure foxes make noise, and of course owls hoot, though Sooki or Kooki never vocalized anything in class. My experience with them has been one of utter quiet.

When I met David Whyte (stay tuned), I saw that he was wearing a Fjalraven jacket. Their items have a fox logo patch sewn onto them. At the time, I had a yellow backpack and a gray wax jacket, which seemed very well-made, and, naturally had the fox emblems. I mentioned the company, questioned David and he seemed surprised

I knew of them. He said they were—are—an excellent company. His daughter-in-law worked for them, their products are of very high quality and they are very socially-conscientious—practiced respect for their workers, for the environment. And of course, since then, and since seeing the fox, I now have Fjalraven fox socks, and shirt, and pants… I even did a hike-a-thon to support nature—and earn a Fjalraven gift card.

My friend, Jason Baker, who is the curator of Red Butte Gardens—another thing that seems impossible and wonderful—I am friends with the curator of a botanical garden!—told me of a park in Murray, a suburb of Salt Lake City, that is frequented by foxes. Actually, at first he did not tell me. Nor—what would have been even better for me—did he draw a map. But he sent me a text with what looked like a red teardrop on it. It was, I learned later, pinpointing the exact location of the wooded area with foxes on a Google map.

But I could not find it and got lost driving around to dead ends in the area. Finally, I sheepishly emailed Jason, and he, if such a thing is possible in email, laughed heartily and kindly. Then he wrote out and sent directions, drew a map, and took and sent a picture of it. I then found the park, and proceeded to get lost on foot, trying to find the area where the foxes were most likely to be encountered. But, Rockstar and I are good at walking, and it is a safe pandemic activity—and eventually we did find them. There and at the nearby Wheeler farm. I told Jason, with relish, about seeing them at the farm, and at the golf course. Though I only saw one at the golf course, and only saw her twice, and should have given Dr. Hardy credit.

This is definitely not a part of this Animal Interlude. But part of Air Fairy's origin story, maybe. In any case, one morning while making the rounds at Murray Park, Jason's fox park, I realized that the path Rockstar and I were following was just across the lawn from a mental hospital. At least the building had been that in the past. I know because it was one in which my mother had stayed for quite some time following one of her suicide attempts. I was about seven years old then. Now nearly forty, I was filled with horror of that past—of visiting her in the rectangles and squares of that brick brown building. Of seeing her, feeling both that I failed to be a good enough daughter for her to want to be alive, and that I could not be at all bad, had to do and be better—or my badness or inadequacy, my failure would tip her over the edge. I feared not being able to be good, delightful, smart, helpful enough. And also not able to disappear, become Air Fairy, need nothing, ask for nothing. And I wanted her to know that she was loved and needed, wanted her not to try to die, again, and again…

Well. It is there. She was there. I was there. I am there. And I am a doctor, there are things I can do now, I have tools, to help, except... Except there is a new pandemic, a new deadly virus and I know nothing, and fear I will fail, fail to keep my patients alive. But…

I am looking for foxes, and Rockstar is waiting for me to catch up.

Hammock—trap

There is a spider near my hammock—
a thing I despise—hammock, not spider.
Silver-grey, swaying its web first caught my eye
near-equal in size,
hammock and web, slung between trunks
stretched side-by-side.
The spider's silks catch light and flies.
The hammock's soft cotton,
its come-hither sway misses its prey—
me. I cannot give way, sit inside,
climb in and lay back, close my eyes.
Lose my mind. Wrestle back,
focus thoughts, my eyes fighting rest
hypnotic swinging low,
to-and-fro, cradle-calm.
Alarm
swooned in sleep
I might miss a beat, miss a call.
Then what patient might die? Spider eyes meet mine.
Five flies at least, she has trapped

and wrapped fast, packed snacks.
And something larger besides,
with whirring wings body worrying still;
cocooned, unrecognizable,
and at least thrice her size.
Should be food for some time,
I suppose, but don't know
the nutritive value of blood.

Superpowers

As I drive home after work, a familiar mix of shock, gratitude, and guilt swirls—that I live here, in this sycamore-lined, storybook-beautiful, old neighborhood. My precocious five-year-old neighbor, Arthur, is at the end of my driveway, today with his older sister Caroline. She is absorbed in sidewalk art, but he watches me.

"Hi, Melissa," he hollers, as I pull in and get out of the car with Rockstar, who also is five years old. Rock goes with me... essentially everywhere I go—which mostly, now, is work and home.

"Hi, Arthur."

"What is this?" He says, kicking something at the end of the driveway. Staying "socially distant," both of us masked.

"Oh, it's petrified wood."

"What is that? Why is it putrefied?"

"Oh, petrified means it is like rock now."

"So it's a rock."

"Well, sort of, it's sort of like a fossil—a wood fossil-rock, old tree…"

"How did you make it?"

"Oh, I didn't really make it."

“How did you find it?”

“Um, actually they were here when I bought this house.” Amazing, I think: these beautiful petrified wood pieces along the east side of my driveway, amongst rocks and moss, and shade perennials. Also amazing how very little I had to do with them being there—and how lacking my earth-science knowledge and explanation skills…

Later, after watching or listening to the slowly increasing number of reliable, useful sources for pandemic information—STAT, NEJM, JAMA; the University of Utah’s weekly, then biweekly, then daily PULSE updates; the WHO—I search for printable information about petrified wood. I print some out, and include pages to color, and I leave them on the porch next door. When I next see Arthur, he is with Caroline, and she tells me thank you for the pages, and that they are in their “quarantine room” where they will stay for three days, then they will be able to handle them safely.

* * *

One day, a Navajo couple, Anna and Bahe, both with initially very poorly controlled—or, really just not acknowledged or treated—diabetes, are on a telehealth visit. Over the past year or two I have seen them in clinic, and been amazed at changes in eating, how faithful they are with taking their medications and checking their glucose levels, and how much better they seem to feel. Bahe lost a toe due to a non-healing wound and is determined not to let his disease take more from him. Anna and Bahe are not able to do video with their simple phone. Although each has an appointment time, they have me on speaker and take turns or talk at the same time. Sometimes I talk at the same time too, unintentionally—phone conversation skills have always eluded me; it is possible that I have, or had, a telephone phobia. Exposure therapy works. Pandemic positivity.

Anna tells me the reservation is on “lock-down.” She is afraid to go out to walk, and that makes her blood sugar higher. Also, they have limited choices for food, no longer making the 2-hour drive to Walmart every week for fresh fruits and vegetables, chicken, yogurt. Bahe is listing family members who "caught the COVID" and have died. His sister and her husband, and their niece and her husband in Arizona, and several aunties, and their friend's parents.

And, and, and...

I am stunned and horrified. And for an awful moment want to cry, or scream. Then, my doctorly voice says, "I am so so sorry." And "You should go outside to walk. It is safe outside. Just stay a distance away from anyone else and start walking every day. You can wear a mask if you want to."

Is it safe outside? I think so. That seems to be true. At least from an infectious standpoint, with the pandemic. When I used to have clinic days on the reservation, Rockstar and I walked during lunch break, and the "rez dogs" seemed far from safe—though, as usual, Rockstar seemed unfazed, and had he not been aware of my high anxiety, would no doubt have trotted off merrily to play—or be cheerfully slaughtered.

That day driving home, I pass an unmanned pumpkin stand, and realize Halloween is Sunday. In my compulsive twice daily email inbox clearing—looking at the reliable sources, latest updates on virus, treatments, looking at daily case counts, hospital capacity or lack thereof, deaths—I have skimmed subject lines from the Neighborhood Post. Is it okay to trick or treat? Surely not—due to COVID; surely not—because it is Sunday (I live in an area highly influenced by religion). Other posts: surely it is not fair to deny children, already missing school friends, grandparents, so much else, to deprive them of a holiday. The best thing to do is leave things on a table on the porch and have only children in same "pod" go together, in masks and gloves and . . .

I buy some knobby pumpkins, leaving cash, which no one uses now, in the pot. I have ordered spray paint—eco friendly, non-toxic, it advertises—in a rainbow of colors, through Amazon Smiles. I convince myself that using an enormous corporation with questionable business practices, putting people doing the delivery at potential risk if they are not given masks and adequate time to make the drives without sleep deprivation, plus pollution of transportation... I tell myself that I am offsetting that by supporting Utah Physicians for a Healthy Environment, with each purchase I make. I also order organic fruit lollipops and recycled wooden pencils with fun—sort of fun—eco-friendly eraser tops, made by a small company in Canada, not by slave laborers in China. I hope.

I spray-paint the pumpkins except one which I cook, and try to eat the seeds, but mostly make a mess. But I like the warm harvest autumn smell, the red-orange-brown colors of the mess. The other pumpkins are rainbow-colored bumpy orbs with silver stems, in my gardens. On Sunday, I spray-paint some angel wings, from a costume I had for a Singles Halloween Dance activity at church—in another lifetime, before the pandemic. I think maybe I will be Air Fairy.

Air Fairy, recall, is me, or is the invention of my psychologist, Dr. Hardy. Or, perhaps it is more accurate to say he discovered her, Air Fairy, or called her out. I had been seeing Dr. Hardy weekly for years when the pandemic started. With the increased stress, isolation—all that has come with it—he began seeing me twice weekly, though "seeing" me became virtual. He has saved my life many times, or maybe it is that he saved it and does so on an ongoing basis. And I am glad because I want to help my patients and feed Rockstar. Dr. Hardy, who is much older and more tech-savvy than I, helped me test and then improve my very poor computer connection. High speed, a necessity, not only for seeing him but for trying to connect with patients at home and watching PULSE, as it gives updated local information about surge-planning, testing, treatment, staffing, ventilators, case counts… and for COVID webinar updates. At the same time, offline, the pace of the world around me slowed. The neighborhood morning ritual rush of children to school, parents to work, then daytime workers: landscapers, cleaners, renovators; the afternoons of school pick-ups, soccer practices, birthday parties, dinner parties, clubs, concerts—all gone, stopped. Even church became a home-based Zoom event. We went for walks, waved, gardened, sat on porches, watched squirrels and birds.

As the pandemic worsened, I was so grateful for the twice-weekly online appointments with Dr. Hardy. My lists of patients to contact and the information to review sometimes was—well, consuming. I had traumatic memories from med school and early residency—memories of impossible workloads, without resources or knowledge to manage. And I started making a strange sort of humming noise, breathing out, maybe to keep out virus? I honestly don't know—it was worse when more tired or anxious. Sometimes I was not sure if people really existed, seeing everyone in Zoom boxes. Dr. Hardy agreed to let me see him, outside, from a distance, in real life—so I knew he was alive and real. More than anything, I wanted to be a good doctor, to help. I loved my patients and an additional hour of therapy a week seemed to maybe make this just possible, kept me from sinking entirely into fear and strangeness.

Me: "But how could I eat or sleep or goof off or whatever, when there might be something to learn that would save a life? Some studies show that having a primary care doctor who cares makes a huge difference in patient outcomes so…" I did not reveal that I believed—even if my rational brain, my scientist brain knew it was crazy—that as long as I saw or "saw" every patient with COVID, continued to talk to each of them until each case was improving, each patient was out of danger—that they would not die. My patients would not die.

Dr. Hardy: "That is bullshit. That is Air Fairy talking. Air Fairy thinks she doesn't need food or rest, can live on nothing and is superhuman." He sang the last sentence in an airy way.

Less airily, he said, "I will not talk to Air Fairy. I will growl at her." He did. "GRRRRRRR. If Melissa is there and wants to do therapy, I am available."

He saved me. I could not manage this work or life without these appointments. So. Air Fairy was scary and became my Halloween costume.

Rockstar and I walked around the neighborhood, me as Air Fairy carrying a painted pumpkin, wearing painted wings, and Rockstar went as a flamingo. Sort of. In that prior world, pre-pandemic life, I had taken my niece and nephew to the Aviary, at which time we purchased pink flamingo wings, meant to be worn by children or small adults, I suppose—but smashing on Rockstar. We walked around the neighborhood.

"Oh, so cute!" Dead brides and garroted cheerleaders cooed.

"Heh, a bird dog, going hunting?" Sort of creepy middle-aged man.

We stayed more than six feet away from the man. And it all rolled off Rockstar, who seemed to love being out, and especially to love the occasional blown kisses by the spooky-pretty girls.

At my house, I thought at first I would do the table with treats, but was afraid kids would congregate and spread COVID and I would be responsible for their illness—which would spread to their grandparents who would die. So, I stuck the pencils and lollipops far apart all throughout my yard and put a sign on the front door to Keep Socially Distant and Feel Free to take a treat and Happy Halloween!

Arthur chose a purple lollipop, maybe grape. I do not know what his costume was, probably a Marvel character. I have never managed to sit through films. He wore a cape and helmet, but he often wears these, one or the other or both, not just on Halloween. He also was eating a purple ornamental kale.

"What is this?"

"Ornamental kale."

"It is not as good as the mint."

"That is true." We both like peppermint and spearmint best.

"Do you like a purple nurple?" Arthur asked.

"Um. I don't know. I sort of like purple," I said

"But what about purple nurple?"

"I don't know, do you?" I returned.

"What is a purple nurple?" Arthur asked.

"I don't know, you're the one who said it. Maybe you made it up?" I replied.

"No! My dad said purple nurple." He seemed indignant.

"Oh. Well did you ask him what it is?" I asked.

"No." he said.

Another day, I ended up sending another husband-and-wife couple, immigrants from Iraq, to the hospital. My schedule listed "monthly follow-up" as the reason for the wife, Muna's, telehealth visit. She coughed through the entire visit, but through coughing told me how her husband, Nasim, is the one really sick—that he is going to or has just passed out, hard to tell from the interpretation, through the static, the coughing and the fear. With help from staff, I sent them an ambulance. They both had COVID and Nasim was severely hypoxic. Both are really high risk for possibly fatal disease. For some reason, they were taken to different hospitals. Their daughters were likely the source of infection—of course my patients follow my counsel to stay home, mask, distance—but their daughters were in community college, young and otherwise healthy. And they are also likely the source of their parents' connection to the world, since they speak English and have become somewhat accustomed to life here, at least pre-pandemic.

I am notified via Teams that Muna's daughter is on the phone to speak to me. I ask them to get the best number, finish my telehealth visit, and then give her a call.

"Hi, this is Dr. Bentley."

"Oh, hi, doctor, thank you for calling, what to do? We are at hospital, we cannot go in." Then tears.

Doctor speaks: "I will check with your parents' doctors and nurses, do not worry, can you tell me where they are?"

"Yes, Mama Muna is at the University, U of U, and Papa Nasim is at St. Luke's. Mama Muna keeps texting us, but now she is not."

"Thank you so much," I say, "I will call the hospitals now and be sure they are well-cared for, do not worry."

"And then will you call us back, Doctor," she says, and it is more of a statement than a question.

And I will, of course.

*   *   *

The situation is a bit tricky. When I watch the PULSE updates or join webinars, I see the shadows around doctors' eyes, even as they calmly and authoritatively release surge plans, discuss crisis standards of care, plead with us to publicize the importance of mask wearing, distancing. Colleagues, co-residents from prior life—when still in training and before COVID— are now working in the ICU and are exhausted. I have signed up, am on a list of community physicians willing to be called upon to provide relief if needed. I still work full time in the clinic, scheduling visits as telehealth but still seeing patients in person who show up or can't access technology. I have masks, and tests. And I have nights, and my full-time is technically four 10-hour days. So I have Fridays and weekends. To my relief (and shame at the relief), they do not call me.

"This is Dr. Bentley. I care for Nasim in my clinic, as you know he has severe COVID 19 infection, his wife is at another hospital, and I wondered if I could speak to him or give him a message... But in any case wanted to give you my name and number if I can do anything or if there are any questions about his history. And I can also pass along information to his daughters…" There is silence.

"Oh. Thank you so much. Um. His nurse is in another patient room should I go get him?"

"Oh, no," I say, not wanting to force the nurse to doff PPE then suit up again, not wanting to add to work or shortages or exhaustion, or do anything that could lead to spread of illness.

"Could you maybe just deliver this message?"

I do hear from some staff, and speak to some patients. Some are too sick to speak, are on ventilators. But they recover. They get my messages. I am doing all I can, they know that I care. I can tell their treatment teams about their chronic conditions that just might matter and just might be enough to keep them from dying. And it works. None of my patients dies, despite what Dr. Hardy said (bullshit, Air Fairy). Even if I know it isn't logical. What if, just what if... somehow—if there's any chance I am keeping someone alive then I just—just have to do it. Air Fairy can work, maybe. It's a new virus, who knows? What else do I do that matters anyway?

* * *

For Thanksgiving, Arthur tells me, they did a Zoom feast with their several Zoom-screens-worth of squares of cousins who live back East.

"My favorite cousin is seven and he lives in New Jersey," he says.

"Oh," I say.

It is unseasonably warm and dry, no snow, and I am raking leaves and putting them in the yard waste bin. Caroline is roller blading.

"You are getting really good at that!" I call.

"What about me?" Arthur asks.

"Um…" He is standing on the side of their tipped-over yard waste bin. Helmet is on.

"You are getting really good at that too," I say.

"At what?" he asks.

"Standing on the bin?" I stammer-ask.

"Yes. Thank you, I really am." Then he asks, "Guess what my favorite cousin's name is?"

"I don't know," I reply.

them and entered things. Most of them could recall no medications they had been prescribed, except occasionally one remembered Lortab or Ativan. These seemed to be top in Rodney's armament, and my suggesting they were not the only or the best options for pain, sleep, anxiety—was not always welcome. The patients felt helped by these medications, and were not so concerned about side effects, addiction, long term problems. When a patient, a person, is in pain, or unable to sleep or relax, has personal and intergenerational trauma, loss, fear—immediate relief is of paramount importance.

Inexplicably, one day when I arrived, the closet-room that I used as my office was stuffed full of—well, stuff. Stacks of large binders, posters, possibly suture or bandaging material, PVC pipe, plastic tubing, and other miscellaneous pieces of plastic, toys, tarps, bottles, light fixtures. In any case, there was no longer a desk or chair, both I assumed buried with the stuff, or moved elsewhere. And though many days there were no patients for hours, this day there was someone already in the exam room and two in the waiting room—possibly three. One of them was a child. As an internist, I do not see children, but as Chris Payne had reminded me, I work for the Tribe—and if I am on the reservation doing the best I can—suturing up a lacerated child's hand, to keep her from losing her finger, ordering an antibiotic to keep "strep throat" from becoming rheumatic fever—well, I will not be faulted or sued if it isn't done perfectly.

Unsure what to do, I used the only available space—the bathroom. In the trailer-clinic, which was tiny, there were, nonetheless, two bathrooms: one adjacent to the patient waiting room, and the other adjacent to the exam room and closet-office. I set my laptop on the sink, using a box lid to create a flat surface to place it upon, and I attached a skeptical-seeming Rockstar to the metal toilet paper cylinder meant to hold toilet paper. It was not a great day. I did my best to love and help the people. But I felt—well, less deserving of space than PVC pipes and discarded pieces of plastic, my work of very little value to the Tribe. I told Chris I needed a desk and chair if I was to go out there again. Maybe that is overly demanding or self-centered. I did work for the tribe, it's true.

One very muddy day, Rockstar and I got into the car to head back to the city, somewhat dreading the long drive, thinking a bit about the few patients I had seen and tried to help, but also thinking of how to stay awake. At our lunch break, Rock and I had gone for a walk and been chased, sort of, by reservation dogs. Their territory, fair enough. They kept just far enough away that I didn't panic, but it was a very brisk return to the clinic trailer. It was mucky anyway, my shoes mud cakes, I tried to clean them off before going back to work and before getting into my car.

As I got in and tried to back up, tried to go—well, I didn't go anywhere, except perhaps down—stuck, sunk into mud-sludge. My tires spun and my bright blue car turned brown and sunk deeper.

Weary, trying not to cry, I got out. I found a shovel and dug around each tire. I found a stick, then more sticks, pebbles, a tarp—. I somehow made a sort of mat or surface for traction. I pushed, prayed, tried backing out again, then going forward... and ultimately got out and got on the road before dark. I know that there were tribal members there, the school and day care were nearby, the offices, homes. They did not come out. The sun was setting behind me, beautiful, and looking very like the sunrise had in the morning, on my way out to clinic. Had it really been just one day? I turned on the radio and happened to catch the tail end of a song, and the station's DJ identified Pearl Jam as the band. I thought of Nick, and my merry library tribe from so long ago. I wondered what had happened to them. I wanted to know—or, rather, I wanted to know that they were happy. I imagined Nick had indeed gone to Notre Dame—family money could make things happen—even if he had spent his school days buying cassettes and vying for the attention of a driven, scared, girl—me. I would like to thank him—to thank them all for—for liking me, for saving me, for not letting me be alone. I did not fit—did not fit in, but I was determined to offer my care, to keep trying to heal or help, to work for the Tribe.

Dear Life

"Blessed are the pure in heart, for they shall see God." Matthew 5:8

As I listen to Jack, I marvel at the way his black skin glows, his brown speckled eyes sparkle. He was hit by a car in his 20s, back broken. He has smoked since he was nine, and cancer led to the loss of half a lung. The remaining lung lobes are scarred, hollowed out by emphysema. He cackle-laughs as he tells me his oxygen was turned down from three liters to two—meaning that he needs less supplemental oxygen than usual to maintain appropriate saturation on his pulse oximetery, 90%. He is combing his hair, and the gray-white curlicue looks like a halo. He lives at a care center, and he has COVID. A death sentence scenario for so many.

We are meeting virtually. I examine him on a screen, available senses limited to sight and sound, unable to touch my patient, to lay on hands. Or to smell or taste, though taste at least I rarely use—maybe good doctors still smell or taste their diabetic patients' urine, to detect ketones or glucose, but… it is possible to smell ketones on the breath too, or to smell the sweet sick rotting smell indicative of a pseudomonas bacterial infection.

To both of our surprise and delight, Jack has not died of COVID; on the contrary for some reason he seems to be thriving. The fear of death, or the joy at not dying, seems to have brought to mind past loves: for poetry writing and for a sister in California, with whom he now has nightly chats. Yet half the staff and unrevealed numbers of patients at Maple Ridge have COVID. Jack's eyes tear up as he tells me of friends who have died. The woman across the hall. The man next door.

"How does my hair look, Doc?" he asks.

"It looks like a halo," I reply.

He cackles. "I will have to tell that to God. He will get a kick out of it."

"Do you talk to God?" I ask, hoping the uneasiness I feel is not in my voice. (Is this delirium?)

"Every night," he replies.

"Does He talk to you every night?" I ask.

"Of course not. What do you think, I'm the Pope?"

No, I do not think that.

"He sometimes gives me messages. And I saw him once," Jack says.

"You saw Him? What does He look like?" I ask.

"A blue jay," he replies.

"A blue jay?"

"It was a long time ago. You know my dad was shot dead before I was three years old. My momma raised me and my sisters, but she caught the cancer, and I didn't see her for a while, then my aunties told me she died, and I ran away. I didn't ever want to be in our house again. I'd make my own way. I ran as long as I could, then I had no breath and sat down on a bench. That is when God came. He sat by me and told me I'd better get myself clean and sober and get myself back home to take care of my sisters. That was my duty. That blue jay God was no squawking bird. He told me that as I am talking to you. I've never seen Him again. But every time I see or hear a jay, it's a good reminder."

And I agree—or rather, I think it is possible to see God in the natural world, experience awe, wonder; and it is easy to forget—to look, to overlook, to travel along in thought without noticing. One of the many unsettling aspects of the pandemic, for me, has been the juxtaposition of the gorgeous Spring, the cherry and crab-apple blossoms, the red-winged blackbirds, the green beneath melting snow, the warm rain and rainbows. But, then—then so many sick patients. And I was their doctor. And scared and…

* * *

Another day during this time, I met with Jimmy, a member of the Choctaw Nation from Oklahoma, now living here in Salt Lake City where he came to be with, and then to marry, his husband. Who has since left him.

I see Jimmy in the square of my computer screen. Somehow the defined space seems to distill or clarify, diminish distractions. The noise of medical assistants laughing or a newly-vaccinated child crying; endless clinic construction noise, somehow ongoing mid-pandemic; phone calls into my office—a request from the pharmacy, a call from an outside physician regarding a mutual patient—all are shut out for now. Things have slowed down, patients and staff in-clinic are minimized, and when I am "with" a virtual patient I am not accessible to anyone else. Even the patient's cell phone going off—this can't happen—he only has one phone and is using it for our appointment, to talk to me, see me. Maybe telemedicine is a sixth sense, to make up for the loss of the other three, somehow. Maybe.

We were scheduled to meet, Jimmy and I, to discuss his diabetes. It has been poorly controlled, which is especially problematic since he has had a prior heart attack, has poor and worsening kidney function, and the elevated blood sugars increase his risk for further vascular disease—another heart attack, or stroke, progressive diminishment of his kidney capacity, ultimately dialysis. He also has had one toe amputated, an unhealable sore—it started as a stubbed toe, but with his vascular disease, inadequate blood supply made it impossible to heal.

All of this he knows. We go over it anyway, each visit. I ask him to bring—or, on video, to hold up—a record with his blood sugar, checked each morning before he eats. I go over each medication, insulin and pills, check the amounts. When he comes to clinic, I check his bag from our pharmacy to be sure that he actually has them. I anticipate doing the same thing online with him today, looking at his pill bottles, asking for his numbers, his questions. He will even be able to show me where he stores his medications, where he takes them. He might be willing to show me inside his kitchen cupboards, his refrigerator/freezer, so I can look for fruits and vegetables, yogurt, fish, nuts… or leftover Chinese take-out, frozen pizzas, ice cream sandwiches.

Today, he is on a new iPad; he seems more adept with technology than I, in some ways, his camera picture is clear, the angle, the focus. His microphone or sound system is clear as well. I struggle with my headphones, adjust the view, try to be able to see his chart and his face and then... Then I stop finicking and look at him.

I watch as Jimmy's beloved cat is having kittens, and as he, Jimmy, is having a heart attack. He is sweaty, hand on chest, telling me he is okay, a bit winded, sort of, well, sore… but the kittens. I am horrified. I cannot touch him, clear as his image is, I cannot use my stethoscope, my hands to feel his pulse, my tools to check his vitals. All I have is my voice and, I hope, my authority, white coat, the diplomas behind me. I also have our history, a track record, our visits, our time together. He knows that I care and have not steered him wrong. He has told me this. I tell him he needs to go to the hospital now, he is having a heart attack. His cat can take care of her own.

Jimmy is so soft-hearted. I couldn't care less about his kittens. Had it been a dog, I might have felt otherwise, but… Soft-hearted, if he has any heart still alive, I think. Any pieces of that tender heart muscle that still has blood supply not blocked by years of diabetes, is set off by genetics, then by displacement into an environment of convenience store food, non-existent or sedentary work, and tobacco.

He does go. When the ambulance I send arrives, he makes it to the hospital in time to have his heart arteries opened, stented.

The next day, there is a gap in my schedule, a previously arranged telehealth visit for a patient now in-hospital didn't get canceled, so I use the time to call Jimmy at the hospital. He doesn't answer, and I leave a brief message. Which is okay, I have learned, since he identifies himself on his voice mail greeting—privacy compliant. Otherwise, it is a HIPAA violation to leave a message. I tell him I will be sure to see him as soon as he is discharged. Strangely, some patients have done virtual visits with me when they have been in hospital, but as regulations have been clarified regarding telehealth, we learn this is not billable. I can do a visit with a patient in a care center, rehab facility, assisted living, but not an inpatient in a hospital. So, I call on my own time and put a "telephone encounter" into the chart if anything needs to be documented.

At our next visit, two weeks later, virtually, Jimmy tells me that his landlady cared for his cat. One kitten didn't make it. Still, Jimmy is grateful to be alive. And he resents not being able to save that one. He has a sort of memorial service, though the landlady put the body out with the trash. He would like to have buried him/her properly.

"But still, thanks anyway, Doc. I guess my heart is cleaned out and pure again," he says.

And so, we are back to our usual visit duties. We try to sort through what medicines he is taking, he has a plastic Walmart bag full of bottles, and I have an electronic copy of the hospital discharge summary with a medication list. He holds up each bottle so that I can see the label on his iPad, and we try to reconcile the two—the medications on the list and the medications in his bag. Hospital stays always wreak havoc on tidy medication lists. I tell him which medicines he should restart—ones they ought not to have stopped, and I tell him to stop the ones they started that might not be needed. It is a process made more difficult by the plethora of cats, streaking across the screen to attack his plastic bag, then batting around the medicine bottles. I pray they do not come open, I do not want to watch him pick up each tablet or capsule, show it to me for identification, put it back in the right bottle, keeping his cats from eating any pills, me worried about his activity, balance, heart…

"Well. I am glad you are alive. Sorry about your kitten," I say.

"Not my time yet, maybe God wants me to take care of these cats first," he says. "And I am happy to oblige. Not ready to die. I tried that before."

"You did?" I ask.

"But God stopped me," he replies.

"He did?" I ask. "Did he look like a blue jay?"

Jimmy looks at me with complete incomprehension.

"A blue jay? No, Doc, He's an old man with a shiny white head of long hair, and a beard. He smells like rain and trees and oranges. Not that you asked," he says.

"Tell me more," I say.

"It was a long time ago. Back home, on the Rez. Kids were teasing me because I wouldn't go hunting and other things so—well they called me homo—they could tell—and I was—and I was ashamed but at last confessed at Sunday school, and then Pastor told me I was a sinner, that anytime I felt love for a man I was hurting God. But I couldn't help it, I couldn't stop. Loving, wanting. And I didn't want to hurt God. So, I took that hunting rifle and went off into the trees, deciding that was the only way I could stop hurting God." His usually open, smiling, ruddy face looks suddenly solemn, taught-jawed, determined.

"To kill yourself?" I ask, stunned. He nods on the screen.

"But that is when God came. I felt someone behind me and I turned and He was there. He took the gun from me. He breathed on the back of my neck. And it was love and life, He loved me and wanted me to live and to love. I saw the tree leaves around us trembling, and the water on the pond sort of moving, the top skimmed with His breath, and then I felt His breath through my whole body and mind."

"Did you see Him again?" I want him to say yes, that his whole hard life God has been with him, buoying him up, life-affirming, soothing.

"No. He was gone when I turned around. But it's my duty now to live and to love. And all these cats…"

I say with what I hope is some sincerity that, unfortunately, I am allergic and cannot provide a forever home to any of them. He knows my dog, Rockstar, from pre-pandemic days when he met him in clinic, and so he may not have tried to give one to me anyway.

*   *   *

And I want God to be there in the breeze or the birds, or the computer keys, screens, somewhere, as another day I meet, virtually, with Eliza, who is dying. And my heart is breaking. She used to live in a downtown apartment near my clinic, but now stays with an adult daughter in Provo, about 60 miles south of Salt Lake City. Eliza has cholangiocarcinoma, a bile duct cancer, widely metastatic, but held in check for some time. By "held in check" I mean beaten back with surgery to remove the largest masses, chemotherapy to try to poison the tumors without completely poisoning every one of her healthy cells, and radiation—again to try to destroy more of the cancer and spare her other parts when able. She is seventy-five, and I sense that were it not for the cancer, she would have been decidedly spry, her eyes and smile still those of someone 20 years younger. She sports various wigs, or goes baldish, short hair spikes dyed lavender, matching lipstick.

"Hi," I say, as she appears on my screen, her daughter, Bonnie, having answered the phone, just as I was about to give up, the tenth ring. Bonnie looks fresh from a shower, face ruddy, wearing a thrown-on towel. She got her mother, set up the video, then left the screen with a screaming child in tow.

"Well," Eliza says. "I have to tell you, I found a jack fruit at the store, Bonnie took me in a wheelchair, which is fine, I could walk, but she wanted to do the chair, so I let her…"

She tells me of the many virtues of jack fruit and how much the B12 shots I give her help her, how she feels like dancing for a few days after a shot.

"I'm so glad it helped and glad to know that about jack fruit, too," I say. "I am sorry, but please don't dance. Be careful…"

Her very osteoporotic bones will splinter. I think for some reason of Ezekiel, the dry-bones. God, do you see her very dry bones? Lord, hold them together, keep them lively. I think I have that story wrong. All I remember, honestly, is a song about Ezekiel and "them dry bones" and "the head bone's connected to the neck bone, now hear the word of the Lord." Even that I think I have wrong.

Then Eliza is in hospital— I learn this the week after our dancing jack fruit virtual visit. I ask my medical assistant to relay a message to Bonnie, and I get a telephone counter back in my electronic health record that says Bonnie says Eliza is in the hospital and they think she will die. I follow her case remotely, online, scouring imaging reports and progress notes. The cancer has perforated her bowels, they see air in places they should not. But she is started on TPN, total parenteral nutrition, food infused into her veins. She can have nothing to eat or drink by mouth or it would go out the holes in her intestines and cause overwhelming infection, death.

Eliza does not die. The hospital notes from social workers document discussions about possible hospice. But she says she is not ready for that yet. She wants them to do everything. She wants to do everything. To live. She goes back to live with her daughter. And her daughter calls, another telephone encounter in the computer chart, Bonnie wants to schedule her mom to meet with me as soon as possible.

We meet online early, I have had to work her in. I am afraid if I don't, I will not see her again. She is so frail, and my schedule is filled with the sick. I apologize for the early hour. She has put on lipstick and mascara. She is wearing an aquamarine shirt with "*joie de vivre*" written across the front in hot pink script.

"I like your shirt," I say.

She tells me it was on the table—at her prior apartment complex, there was a table in the lobby where residents could leave items or take items. She once brought me a white coat for work, she thought would be a perfect fit, she had been eyeing it for some time, thought it too small for most people.

"Tags still on," she showed me, proudly. Today, she tells me that she loves me, and I say I love her back. I wonder if that is something a doctor ought not to say. She wants to eat. She wants to live. She canceled the colorectal surgery follow-up appointment because she told them she was seeing her primary care doctor, her internal medicine doctor, online, and it's too hard to travel. But how can I repair broken bowels, remove cancer that is now everywhere? If my heart was pure, could I see God, could He show me what I need to see, what I can do, somehow, something? I can order shower chairs and B12 shots through home health and send PT and OT, but…

Or surely Eliza has a pure heart—perhaps she will see God and see a way—but she doesn't want to die, she wants to dance, and I don't want to kill her, her love of life, or her hope, with my lack of skill, or knowledge, or faith. I don't see God. I want to see Eliza. Even framed in my computer screen, even ravaged by cancer, she is beautiful and lively.

Elijah swinging low with his sweet chariot, but Eliza isn't ready to go home.

Training

Friedrich Nietzsche—Beyond Good and Evil: "That which does not kill us makes us stronger."

Mary Oliver—"The Wild Geese": "You do not have to be good... you only have to let the soft animal of your body love what it loves."

Training to be a gymnast and training to be a doctor are strikingly alike. Strength of mind and body, the ability to perform well through pain and fatigue are of paramount importance for success and are highly praiseworthy. The goal is perfection, repeating a move, a twist, a flip, a routine, over and over: abdominal muscles tight, each limb, joint, toe perfectly placed. No errors. In medicine, first do no harm. The necessity is perfection: each order, examination, assessment, procedure. Having been in the gym for three hours or in the hospital for thirty hours are not excuses for mistakes. That time is necessary for conditioning, toning and strengthening muscles and mind, and is a sign of dedication: to the sport, and to the patient, the profession.

Fracture

noun: *the act or process of breaking or the state of being broken especially: the breaking of hard tissue (such as bone)*

verb: *to damage or destroy as if by rupturing to cause great disorder in; to break up: fractionate: to go beyond the limits of (something, such as a rule): violate*

In the gym. A flip, a slip, a fall. A chance to be stronger, to practice through pain. But then a film, an x-ray: I was not strong enough to manage, to keep up in practice. And a diagnosis: a fracture. But concerning, to break, to shatter a bone this way, at only twelve. Still, years pass, I work hard in school, in the gym, I compete in meets, I get into medical school. I fall and break a rib. And then another film, a DEXA bone density scan, and another diagnosis: osteoporosis.

In the classroom and on medical wards. This is a time that I am studying medicine in both. I learn that the diagnosis of osteoporosis is based on standard deviations from expected values for age. There is not enough evidence to use certain scoring systems in younger, theoretically premenopausal, women. But by any standard—Z or T score or the raw density numbers—my bones are osteoporotic, weak, porous, not strong. Risk for fragility fractures. Stress fractures. I have patients with osteoporosis, "little old ladies" with devastating hip fractures, or excruciating vertebral compression or "wedge deformity" fractures. Not me. I read, know, that a most important treatment for osteoporosis, or to keep bones strong in the first place is weight-bearing exercise. I was a gymnast. I run. I loved feeling strong, flying around the uneven bars, up to high school, when the gym time became, as hard as I tried, too much with all I had to do for a scholarship, eventual medical school... And at five-foot-five-inches, I was too tall to be a really good gymnast. Perhaps my excuse for giving it up, for quitting. But now, I love running up and down mountains. Marathons. It has not killed me—so then (Nietzsche) it has made me stronger. Not fragile. Not broken.

Medical strength training: in the hospital. On the wards, on rounds, more than in running or tumbling—jumping, landing, pounding—I feel at risk for fracturing, being fractured.

An attending, Dr. McKellar, for whom it is a matter of pride to make each new intern cry on rounds, preferably in front of patients, by asking questions designed to highlight a trainee's lack of knowledge. He is an oncologist, hematologist, and oncologist. These specialties are one, hematology/oncology, treatment of blood disorders and cancer.

But there are patients with benign blood disorders and there are patients with malignant tumors, and they are not at all the same. I love looking at blood smears, seeing and hearing patients with anemia or clotting problems or bleeding problems, then looking at their blood cells in the microscope, especially if what they have is a recognizable and treatable problem. Hematologic disorders. With cancer, however, the science and paper/lecture learning is compelling, yet seeing such very sick patients, very sick cancer patients, made oh-so-much-sicker by their treatments is gut-wrenching. Among the reasons I ultimately decide not to pursue this sub-specialty.

This evening, I have to tap a pleural effusion, fluid that has accumulated around the lung of a patient with lymphoma. I walk into the patient's room, in the beautiful Huntsman Cancer Hospital, a new hospital at the time, built with so many donations made in honor of loved ones who died of cancer.

"Hello, I'm Dr. Bentley. Ms. Johnson, we are going to drain some of the fluid from around your lung. I think it may help you feel better, make your breathing easier, and we can also test it to be sure you don't have an infection or heart failure or any other problems we need to know about. Is that okay?"

"I have heart failure now too?" she says and starts to cry.

"No, no, you don't, you have lymphoma, and I think that is causing the fluid to build up. I just meant… Anyway, no, I am sorry, I didn't mean to upset you," I hastily say.

"Sorry," she says. "I'm just really tired." Then she vomits.

For a moment I think of asking the nurse to come clean her up before the fluid tap, but I recognize that error before I make it, for once, the nurses' shifts are deadly busy, this is something I can do—and I help the patient get cleaned up, then get her a warm blanket and then I do request her nurse to bring nausea medicine and a cup of ice, when she has a moment. If that doesn't happen by the time I am done, I can go get it.

"Ms. Johnson, can you just lean over the table?" I request, putting her hospital table/tray next to the bed, and helping her sit up with her arms on the table, torso leaning over, so that I can access her ribcage from the back side. "You can put your head down and rest if you like."

The oncology fellow, Luke, has come, and I really wish he would just do the tap. I know I am to learn. But, as happens throughout medical school, residency, I cannot stop the thought, the belief, that it is not fair that my learning could harm a patient. I have asked Luke to do it, outside the patient room. He said, "You'll be fine and I'll be there with you."

I don't feel fine, but he is here with me.

I tap her back with my fingers, percussion, listening for the spot where the resonance over the air-filled lungs becomes dull, the top of the fluid, the effusion. We did not use bedside ultrasound or send her down to radiology. It was late, she was struggling to breathe, so there was some urgency. It was also a matter of pride in the program, the ability to diagnose and treat using physical exam findings: developing skilled diagnosticians and proceduralists. So this is what I had to do to be a good doctor.

I mark the spot on her back, looking to Luke, who nods. I have set up a sterile tray, the iodine swabs, the needle and syringe, the bottles for fluid collection, a Band-Aid. I go in just above the rib, as I have been taught, slide along the edge to avoid the neurovascular bundle and—

There is a scream. It is from my patient. Then she starts to sob. I am horrified. I have no idea what I did wrong. Fortunately, my horror has left me frozen, rather than wildly moving the needle with the possibility of allowing air into the thorax and causing the lung to collapse.

"Are you okay?" I ask, stupidly.

She doesn't answer, just sobs. Quietly now, wetly.

I look to Luke. He shrugs but does take the needle from me. The syringe fills with cloudy fluid. Wordlessly, I connect the tubing and we, or he, drains 1.5 liters, an impossible amount to be surrounding her lung in that space—how fortunate that we have two lungs, I think, again, stupidly.

I have a brief 6 hours at home, having been in the hospital from early in the morning to nearly midnight—to try to sleep, or something, I suppose, eat maybe—what does one do? What do normal people do at home? Then I need to be back to pre-round the next day before rounds with the attending. I am trying not to think about a suffering

Ms. Johnson, suffering I may have somehow made worse, and not to be fearful of the day to come, wanting so much to learn, to be good, a good doctor; hardened, strong, and yet, trying not to be broken beyond repair in the process.

I leave before dawn. It is the edge between autumn and winter, and a deer darts across the highway, possibly displaced by hunters, or too hungry to keep to the mountains. I do not know what to do, as seems so often to be the case. (Fracture: breaking up, great disorder). The deer slams into the windshield with incredible power, my neck snaps back, somehow I keep on the road. I do not stop. My windshield is broken, there is a gaping hole, and the rest of the glass is cracked, a sickeningly beautiful blood-red shatter pattern. I make it to the hospital and park. There is hair or fur, whichever makes up a deer's coat, in the front grille. I feel guilt and disgust and guilt at my disgust, the damage I have done, the mess I've made of a deer, a life.

I see my patients early. Then we meet to begin the endless team rounds. Dr. McKellar is in fine form.

I begin my formal bedside presentation of the case of Ms. Johnson, trying to remember the format preferred by this attending. Brief history of present illness, 24-hour events… I am soon interrupted.

"Dr. Bentley, can you tell us what drugs comprise Ms. Johnson's chemotherapeutic regimen, where she is in planned cycles of this course, and what the likely and most consequential adverse effects of each agent?" Dr. McKellar asks. Some residents would say "pimps" not "asks," but I find that too vulgar. "Pimping interns" is something of a sport amongst certain attendings, and even amongst more senior residents. I am trying somehow to be—what? Hold on to some self that maybe never existed in the first place…

I give him the information, and I do know it. And I should. It matters, it is her life I am trying to save. My patient. I do wish I did not have to list the horrific toxicities of our "care" with her listening. But I do.

"Please list the five named women in the New Testament of the Bible," he then requires.

I am taken aback. He once saw me praying with a patient. Perhaps this is retribution for the unsanctioned procedure.

"Mary, the mother of Jesus, Martha, the other Mary…" my voice trails off.

Ms. Johnson laughs. Dr. McKellar laughs. I try so hard not to cry, I bite down hard on the sugar-free life saver in my mouth, and a front tooth fractures. I cry.

Temple

How making vows, naming the dead, blessing ancestors could be
more than spells or superstition

I confess I do not understand.

Maybe it is not.

Inherited religion, the comfort of culture practiced mid-pandemic—
patterns and prayers as known as those sewn onto Pioneer quilts,
wishing for wrapped warmth.

I hope for faith, and I pray, and the temple spire pierces heaven or
simply points to the miracle blue sky.

I read of intergenerational trauma how horrors long ago are encoded,
genetic modification, sub-cellular scars.

Can rituals undo, decode, can words, water, white robes probe the
depths, open the graves, decrypt, dispel, put hungry ghosts to rest?
Does my bowing here put wrongs to right?

Entombment in a stony sanctuary or spreading solace, calming waves
cold feet on solid sea.

Short Story

Some days I think I will tell Dragon a story—instead of dictating a formatted medical note. To be a storyteller, to give Dragon a saga, a gorgeous gripping tale. To tell a story the way I would tell a bedtime story to April, my soon-to-be-eight-year-old goddaughter, full of fairies, witches, or, yes Dragon, okay—Dragons—knights, princesses, dwarves. To use words like "swashbuckling" and "damsel," "ogre" and "charming" and "enchantment."

Some days, rarely, I feel I would like to sing, rather than dictate. Very rarely I do. (Only in early mornings, when the clinic is otherwise empty). Years ago, maybe another lifetime, before the pandemic when singing in choirs became deadly, I was in one—a choir. It was a church choir, and since I was in it, obviously no audition was required. Despite that, probably due to an amazing director and a few very talented opera singers—it was good. The choir sounded excellent. Other people noted this, we were asked to perform at regional conferences, at cultural events—but also, though not a singer, I could tell. It feels different, being part of a musical group that practices and blends, hits pitches right-on, keeps tempo, matches dynamics—musicianship. We spent time and we paid attention to detail and we all loved and wanted to be there, together, singing. Our voices were both individual and blended.

I want that today, but I do not want to sing.

—It is dark, and it is very cold, which makes me short—short of breath, short-tempered… but I want to feel a part of that choir, part of something beautiful, challenging: singing that lifts and doesn't spread disease. With people, shoulder-to-shoulder and not—not alone.

So, I think, maybe I want to tell Dragon my story. Something. To be not so alone.

Once upon a time, I was born. I was, as they say, an accident. After initially being too cold to stay out of the baby oven and having something wrong that made it so I projectile vomited every time I nursed, I was, I have been told, an exceptionally easy baby. And then for as long as I can remember, I wanted always to be good. So much. My poor, very-young, student parents. I did all I could to obey perfectly, to do perfectly in school. I tried not only to be no bother, but to be wanted, delightful and… well, to at the very least not deepen the difficulties I saw creased into my parents' brows. Unfortunately, I failed. My father disappeared and my mother continually tried to die. My older sister's heart failed, and my baby brother's brain bled, and there was nothing I could do. Helpless and childish.

But, with time, with the help of teachers, with hard work and God's grace, I went to medical school. I became a doctor. I could do something. I could be a doctor for people who needed one. Help. Keep people alive. I love my work and I love my patients and at times it seems some way in which to—well it's probably wrong, but to feel I have some bit of goodness and some bit of power. *Something*.

And yet, I too was ill and have gotten worse and worse (see elsewhere in this book for details; or, since dictating, "the interested reader might refer…"). And then there was a pandemic. Many people died and I did not know what to do… do not know what to do. Well, I do, the only thing I know—I work.

"Wake up," I say to Dragon. "Ms. Steele is a 42-year-old woman with history of diabetes, hypertension, hyperlipidemia, other conditions as detailed previously here with cough and fever…"

Lifeguard

Life. Guard.

A lifeguard stands sentinel
hawk-eyed, muscles taut,
watching me. Guarding my life.

A gift hard to fathom:

that while I am pool-running the Crimson Lagoon, early morning—so early, so often alone, so quiet save the slipping of water, as my pale limbs send slight waves, barely brushing the blue side-tiles, and the soft sound of breath—there is, listening, there is, standing near, this sentinel.

If sitting, his chair is a watchtower, and what he is watching is me.

He is guarding my life. He is strong and skilled, and holds a red rescue tube. A silver whistle glistens on his chest; he can keep me from sinking, from drowning, from death.

I too would like this calling: Lifeguard. Guarding my patients, fighting back death, disease, decay.

I am a doctor, a physician.

Doctor, from Latin: teacher.

Physician, from French: physic—treatment, remedy. So I do prescribing and teaching, but what about guarding, and life? My patients face death, drowning, so sick, unhoused, undocumented,

“underserved,” we say;

poor and frail and afraid.

There is a pandemic.

I need strength and skill, courage, guarding their lives, against virus, loss of breath—

“Be a guardian, self.”

I long for the power of a red rescue tube, to preserve life, to save.

I pull on my white coat. I think of the lifeguard, his vigilance, his searching eyes, his serious mouth. I think of the silver whistle, and place my stethoscope around my neck, enter the clinic, my first patient waiting.

Triage

It is nearing the end of the day. Both the end of the workday and the end of daylight, fall turning into winter, shorter afternoon light. My final two patients are a mother and daughter, from Iraq. They have been in the United States maybe a decade, maybe a bit less. They do not speak English. The daughter has cerebral palsy or an anoxic brain injury, or a severe infection as an infant with high fever, or cystic fibrosis—or maybe a combination of all or some of these… depending on which notes I read, or what the mother says on a given day. They are waiting for me in a clinic room with east-facing windows, the mountains lit by the setting sun. Our clinic building is located in a poor, busy area downtown, and so usually there are people on the streets, or the lawns, and today is no exception. I look out, briefly, as I enter the room and decide where I can stand or sit to keep the greatest distance between myself, the interpreter, and the two patients. When did medicine change from laying on healing hands or the use of physical diagnosis to the keeping of enough distance, masking appropriately, or completely avoiding contact via telehealth? Pandemic work.

My patients are seated: mother in a chair, daughter in a wheelchair. The interpreter stands behind the door, and I enter and close it, wash my hands, take a breath: focus, prepare to listen. The mother tells me she has had fever and body aches for a few days. That is about as much as I take in before stopping her.

"Did you tell that to the nurse in triage?"

"No one stopped me. There was no triage."

Like many or most medical and dental clinics, hospitals, we have set up a barrier where patients enter the building, in order to try to keep people who may have COVID 19 from entering the clinic. Questions such as, have you had a fever, cough, exposure to someone with COVID 19, loss of smell or taste, body aches, recent travel—the exact questions have changed with the course of the pandemic, our understanding of the virus or variants or risk factors. If they pass screening, patients are then allowed into the waiting room area, the pharmacy, other parts of the clinic. If not, a physician or physician's assistant or nurse practitioner is asked to assess the patient, and, if we have testing supplies, we can test them—or they are advised to go to an urgent care or elsewhere.

For some reason, this barrier—in our case a table with a nurse and a security person—has come to be called "triage." Triage, as a noun, refers to the process of determining which patients are the sickest and require care most urgently, a way to allocate resources. Triage as a verb is the process of doing this, triaging. Somehow our screening patients and then keeping them out if they are likely to be sick and to spread illness to others doesn't seem to fit this definition. But it is necessary, this process, whatever we call it, in a deadly viral pandemic.

So. My patient has fever, body aches…

"Did you tell that to the nurse in triage?"

"They didn't stop me. No triage, they did not ask anything."

So, I walk out to triage. The nurse sitting there tells me that she did indeed stop this mother and daughter and that they denied any of the concerning symptoms or history—they passed. The nurse does not speak Arabic and the patients do not speak English, so I press a bit—she shows me a card that she hands to them, written in Arabic, with the questions, to which they then reply.

I am a little weary and remind myself to focus on the patient. Patients. These particular patients. It must be so difficult to be in a foreign country, to have fled one's homeland and arrived—only to not speak the language and to have a disabled child and, today, to be stopped at triage and presented with screening questions. They arrived on our clinic transport van, large enough to accommodate the daughter's wheelchair. She does not speak. She likely aspirates chronically. She has seizures. It is difficult to keep her masked. The screening questions are written in Arabic, but not all patients can read. All of this in a jumble in my mind, facts and attempted understanding, and compassion, and looking for a breakdown in the system, gaps through which illness slips.

When I go back into the room, having reviewed vital signs and spoken with my medical assistant, I realize that the mother has had fever and night sweats for 4 days and was not tested for COVID. Her chief complaints, reason for visit, are rash and need for me to do disability paperwork; and stomach pain; and depression and fatigue; and body aches and allergies and...

As I listen, the mother reports symptoms of fever off and on for a few days. She also says she and her daughter were recently at the hospital emergency room. The daughter was seen, but not tested for COVID: she was thought to have cellulitis and started on an antibiotic. The mother was tired of waiting to be seen, so left without being evaluated herself, in the emergency room. Emergency departments and hospitals are beyond capacity with patients waiting hours and hours, days...

In any case. Of course I order COVID testing for the mother, who is positive, and then her daughter. In the meantime, she has asked about paperwork for disability, and the proper diapers for her daughter, not the low quality ones, and they must be delivered to her, and she has taken too much allergy medicine due to rashes and is out, and has not been to the allergist because she doesn't have a ride and she… The daughter has COVID 19 as well.

"Why did you lie in triage?" I ask. I probably could have been more diplomatic.

She then calls her son. Who is also my patient. With a full practice, closed to new patients, theoretically—I only take new patients if—well really if my other patients ask me—and so I am fortunate to see extended families. The way they interact is often revealing and puts health and illness into a context that makes some sense of what might otherwise be just frustrating at times, or labeled "noncompliance." In this particular case, the son is my patient, and has been in Turkey to have surgery done, much more quickly and less expensively than would have been possible here—and because of this, the mother has not been able to rely upon her son for transportation. To the allergist, for instance. Or to pick up diapers. The grandparents in the family are also my patients and, fortunately, after extended discussions on several occasions, they are vaccinated. I am hopeful that they will not get COVID or will have mild cases if they do.

I do not know what the mother is saying to her son, or why she called him, exactly. My interpreter is gone. She left as soon as she knew we were testing for COVID. I find out later that this interpreter—who is so skilled, my first choice always—is unvaccinated "for religious reasons," though she is Muslim, and the most devout Muslim patients I see, and staff, are vaccinated, I think. And she has been with me as patients have described vaccine fears, heard my sometimes—though clearly not always—convincing explanations, recommendations for taking the vaccine. She has heard me tell of patients and staff who have died of COVID, has listened as patients relate going to the Middle East to mourn, an older brother, a parent, who died of

COVID, funeral long delayed due to the pandemic…

And so. I am there. Here. In the clinic room. Darkness growing outside. I look at the daughter. She is smiling at me. Maskless. Bad teeth, she refuses brushing and dental care. My heart, my chest feels tight. Her lungs are so raspy at the best of times, and she can't cough well and she doesn't eat well and—and for whatever reason, she is so dear—so much character in her grin, in the noise she makes at times, and I am worried…

And then, for a moment, I am also angry. This woman has exposed my staff, and they are scared, and she has delayed diagnosis and treatment for her daughter. She should have given her symptoms when she made the appointment, and if not that, then at least told the triage nurse so I could go out to meet them in the foyer and plan. The transportation staff did not wear masks, and are also scared, refusing to transport the patients now. Fortunately, the clinic is mostly empty—vulnerable patients may have been exposed as well.

And then again anger is replaced by concern—about the daughter. She cannot cough well. She may die, I think. And the mother, too, is high risk—has diabetes, obesity, is elderly—actually not the case, as I look at her age again—she is just a bit older than I am, is not yet fifty—young for my patient population—but somehow she gives the impression of age…

During the pandemic, some have called health care workers heroes. I am not the least bit heroic, but am sort of angry and scared and maximal OCD. But people helped me that evening, heroically. A medical assistant who speaks Arabic stayed and interpreted for me, relaying information to the patient, getting an oximeter, translating my advice regarding symptomatic treatment, quarantine/isolation, when to go to the hospital—and she also started contact tracing. Another staff member helped me arrange alternate transportation to get them home, and then, after I set up monoclonal antibody treatment, made sure they were able to get to that the next morning. Staff helped get them their prescriptions, wheeled them to the van that would then transport them home. All heroes.

Another definition I came across for "triage" involves a "chance for survival."

* * *

In the morning of this day, which seems weeks ago, on my way into clinic, I had sort of stepped on someone. The secured parking garage has a one-way iron door leading to some cement steps that then lead to the clinic. It is complicated, but my fob allows me to enter the garage, then there is an unlocked door leading to the stairs, but when it closes behind me it is then locked—I can't go backwards through it. On a landing inside that door, something was blocking the stairs, and only after trying to move the something away from the door, did I realize it was a blanket with a man inside. My dog, Rockstar, accompanies me to work, and was on a leash on the other side of the door. He had held back, behind me, as I pushed my way through the door, and now I could not get back out. I was afraid the man was sick or dead, yet not only or even primarily because that would be sad—but he was in my way, and I had so much to do, to try to be ready for the complicated work with patients that lay ahead—and now with my dog on the other side, and I couldn't get back to him and… and if this man was sick I would have to figure out what to do and if dead, figure out what to do then and find someone to help and no one was there and… this, my inconvenience—paramount in my mind—not this man's life. I even saw him as—well, I saw a blanket and then realized there was a man inside, and I wished it was just a blanket—things are just so hard when people are involved.

Fortunately, I suppose, he seemed possibly drugged or drunken or ill or even dead. He just said he was "waiting for Gino," and moved aside. I told him my dog wasn't able to get through.

"Beautiful dog," he mumbled, slurred.

"Thank you," I said automatically. "But…"

The man said he'd watch him—which worried me, but he couldn't get to my dog either… So I ran up the stairs, then back outside, then back into the garage using my fob, then got Rockstar, then got us both into the building then into my office—and was exhausted before the day started. If that man had been sick, would I have helped him: the sickest, possibly dying person, triage? Or would the need to hold together, keep some sort of schedule and order, in order to be able to help the most patients I could be my priority, to stay focused, sterile, to keep chaos from killing, disorder, disease…

*   *   *

After the mother and daughter and staff are gone, I am in my office with Rockstar. I let him out of his kennel. When I look over at him, during the days, usually he appears to be laughing at me.

Understandable. And helpful.

"Wake up."

My Dragon microphone icon turns from yellow and slanted, as it is when "sleeping" in my monitor taskbar, to green, upright, and ready. And I start to tell it about this "patient encounter" making sure to include time spent, for billing purposes. I have taught Dragon commands, Macros that allow me to insert text I use often by using only one word—the command. This one is "Dragon" and when I say that, text appears: a disclaimer about the note being done using Dragon dictation and that any errors are its fault, not mine—which seems a bit unkind, I suppose, blaming the very helpful programmed creature…

And then I leave too, scanning stairwells—no blankets or bodies—tired, hungry, but feeling that that is the only way to manage: *Air Fairy*, yes, Dr. Hardy. Be tough, and the chaos all around and the unmanageable possibly life-threatening situations over which I have no control, but for which I bear responsibility—they can just be about navigated with Air Fairy's help. Maybe. Only not. I am really, really tired. And this strategy learned in med school, or residency, or as a gymnast, or in childhood—

Well. That is another story, and though I sometimes put off going to bed, because then it will be the next day, and I may not know what to do or be able to do it—for tonight, Rockstar and Air Fairy plan to rest.

Roots. Uprooted

I watch the white-blond curls bobbing, swirling, shivering as my goddaughter, six-year-old April, dances through the snake spit fountain.

Long ago, a million years or close to forty, my hair, now the brown-blonde-gray it turned in medical school, was that same blazing light gold. I hear April's laugh, bubbling with the water of the fountain, and the sound, the sun, the grape Jolly Rancher smell of the variegated irises combined are mesmerizing, my eyes close for a moment. Breathe. I open my eyes and see no child.

"April!" I call, still the faintest child laughter, hers, though maybe just echoing in my ears.

"April!"

I am nearly sure she has gone into the garden tunnels, the wonderful maze of totally-enclosed vine-covered trellises that swirl through the Children's Garden. They are tall enough that I barely have to duck to enter, but I'm afraid if I do, I'll choose the wrong path and April will get farther and farther away. She is my brother's daughter, my niece, as well as my goddaughter.

Rather than enter the tunnels, I find a high place, atop a lizard statue, I realize, from where I can look down onto the trellis maze, see each possible entrance and exit. And then the flash of those white gold locks emerges, and I swoop down to scoop up the laughing, fountain-wet little girl and hold her close a moment, until she squirms away, grabs my hand and

"Auntie M, come on!" drags me back to the snakes, insisting that I dance with her in their freezing cold spit.

Dr. Hardy has urged me to take my role as godmother seriously, and heaven knows this child is dear to my heart, I would do most anything, I think, to keep her from harm. I have insisted on learning before play, here at the Botanical Gardens, and have shown her the plant signs, created, I know, by my friend Jason, who is the plant curator. The symbols, I tell her, show you which are water-wise, those have a raindrop that is almost entirely empty; those that need more water have the drop more colored-in. The sun means they need sun; the partial sun or cloud means shade-tolerant, or shade-loving. And so on. This much I can teach. Although monthly I take a class with Jason teaching, "101 Plants to Know" I seem to learn and forget each class, so that I am possibly perpetually learning the same 101 Plants—and happily. It doesn't really matter. Unlike my work as an internist with incredibly complicated, poor, homeless, refugee, Native American, or just old and frail patients, work in which a mistake, something forgotten could, literally, be fatal—here it doesn't matter—I can forget the characteristics of the Aster family, or the difference between the native and non-native Oregon Grape, and no one dies. And I can remember little bits, how Arrowleaf Balsam root smells like chocolate milk powder, and Voodoo Lily smells like rotting meat. Or I can forget and learn again.

I wrap April in my fleece pullover, and again pull her close, trying to absorb her heat, inhale her child smell. There is the slightest breeze and I am freezing. Again she wriggles away, laughing as she runs ahead towards the gates, and I hurry to keep up, afraid she will trip;

her knees, just visible below the hem of the pullover are already scabbed, and I don't want them to scrape off, hurt, bleed. I love these Fridays with her. I don't have clinic, and can usually figure a way to spend a few hours with April, fitting into her parents' schedules or lack thereof, and arranging the time around my standing appointment with Dr. Hardy, and some smattering of other necessary things, medical appointments, dental work, home maintenance, dog training, etc.

As a gymnast, a runner, an always-outdoor child myself, I was perpetually scraped, broken, bruised. Perhaps I was not careful enough, careless, though not carefree. I cared a great deal about following the rules, doing the right things, not causing harm. One morning in the bathroom, I climbed onto the vanity/sink to replace a lightbulb, one of six round glass globes, trying to be helpful, and keep order. I kneeled on my mother's curling iron, which I hadn't realized was plugged in and turned on. Her morning work-readying always involved hair curling and makeup. The skin of my knee burnt. It hurt, blistered and smelled—like burnt flesh, naturally. My mother seemed upset, I wiped off the curling iron, but she wailed "Oh, you will have a scar, your lovely legs will be scarred."

I assured her it was okay. It was not something about which I would have thought to worry.

Scars don't hurt.

I want somehow to know, to feel I have a "place in the family of things," as Mary Oliver wrote, again in her poem "The Wild Geese." Both of my grandmothers have died. My mother's mother died two years before the pandemic, at the end of Spring. My mother had recently visited the cemetery where her grandparents, my grandma's parents, were buried, and she asked them why they didn't come take Leona—my mother's mother. She had dementia, and my mother did not get on well with her.

Perhaps a year before her mother died, my mother moved my grandmother into a care center, closer to her house, and she hired my sister, using my grandmother's money, to help her get ready each morning, set up her pills, and so on. She was too well, my grandma, to need home health, did not qualify for Medicare to cover it based upon her ability to complete ADLs. My grandma was so proud of having paid for her home. She worked her whole life, the only one amongst her siblings to attend college for a few years, and she became a secretary to work for Hercules, an aerospace manufacturing company west of Salt Lake City, for decades. After retirement, she worked for the Church of Jesus Christ of Latter-Day Saints, or Mormon Church in their genealogy/family history efforts, reviewing old documents and entering records into the computer data base, linking ancestors and descendants, creating family trees. When her mind no longer allowed for this, she continued to go for a while, unaware that her work wasn't able to be used, but enjoying or relying upon the routine, familiar routes and people. Her years of work, every day taking a bath, putting on her girdle, curling her red hair. Maybe my mom learned from her, the daily hair-curling. Something I have failed to carry on. But my proper grandmother, putting on a knee-length skirt, ironed blouse, jacket, beige nylons and heels and working every day, allowed her to purchase a home.

When my mother, an only child, was young, my grandma's husband left her—a complicated sad story—so the two of them lived with my grandma's parents. Later, she rented, always working. Finally, when I was perhaps ten years old, she purchased a two-level home in Kearns, one of many growing suburbs west of Salt Lake. She made payments every month, for 20 years. She would tell me how much she still owed, she counted the years, then months then weeks and days until finally she would own her home. In the back yard, she had weeds. But, also, sometimes strawberries. She put down black paper/ fabric to kill the weeds, purchased various gardening tools, and went to work, clearing a space, planting her favorite fruit, strawberries, with which she made freezer jam. She kept it in washed-out cottage cheese containers, saved from her weekly delivery from Winder Dairy. She also washed out the milk and orange juice cartons, all delivered in a silver box on her front doorstep, and made Crystal Lite, strawberry-orange-banana, or mixed berry, or fruit punch. She always said that even when things were very tight, or the situation uncertain, when my mother was small, she could always count on the weekly Winder Dairy delivery. She poured me a glass of orange juice in a very small glass. The glass was thick and flower patterned. I don't drink juice, but I love those glasses, they are in the front of my glass-fronted cabinets, in my own home, on which I make monthly payments.

Along the back of the house my grandmother had roses, inherited from her father, moved from his house; he knew how to grow roses. They were old roses, the ones that smell amazing and are not perfectly shaped, they are leggy or leafy or shrubby. But the smell was the thing, strong, sweeter than anything imaginable, yet not nauseating, just summer and beauty, and gorgeous gobs of petals littering the grass, and the driveway. When my grandmother was living in the care center, Holiday Senior Living, I went back to her home and tried to take a cutting. This was before my mother sold her house, of course. I tried to save those roses, an heirloom, of sorts, an inheritance. I did not really know how, and they died.

Recently, Jason, he of the Botanical Gardens, showed me an incredible technique. He got a 3-D printer, something I never seem to fully grasp. He has used it to make round hollow balls, spheres, which open into two halves. Like those plastic Easter eggs, only perfectly round. For propagation or grafting, he cuts into and peels off the very outer part of a stem, say a rose stem. He makes a slit the length of the diameter of his hollow sphere, and peels around the stem, the outer layer of that portion. He then fills the sphere with rooting material, it looks like dirt, then fits the sphere around the peeled stem and closes it, so that on either end the normal rose stem juts out, and inside the rooting-material-filled sphere there is the skinless bit. After a while, he goes back and opens the sphere and it is full of roots, bursting to be let out. He cuts the stem, and then has the roots to plant, or to graft onto something else.

But back then, I did not know how to do this. My cuttings died, those I tried to plant, those I kept in water and those I tried to graft; I had no idea what I was doing. My mother saw them, the dead stems, and went back to my grandmother's now-sold house. The new owners had not moved in yet, and she dug up several of the roses. I don't know if she replaced them. I don't go to my grandmother's house now, of course, with her not here. I don't know if it seems better, knowing they are in my mother's back yard, assuming they have survived and not been replaced in landscaping, remodeling. Possibly.

My dad's mother, Virginia Sue Johnson Bentley, died either on All Hallows Eve or All Saints Day. She too was at a care center, and the exact time she went from sleeping to dead is not certain, though, as I know, having had to declare patients' deaths during night shifts—called to a bedside, listened for heart beats, touched a glassy eye, checked oculomotor or "doll's eyes" reflex—we do give a time, a time is listed. I think they decided it was still Halloween. She did not die of COVID, though it did enter her care center, isolating her even more, for weeks and months. I read recently that the mortality rate of COVID amongst nursing home residents was approximately 25%. I do not know of what she died, though of course I asked. Maybe she had an infection, that seemed to be part of the problem—but then antibiotics could have been given?

She was not that old, she seemed to enjoy people, chocolates, attention.

With both of my grandmothers, it seemed those around them who were in position to decide, decided that it was time for them to die. Perhaps they would have said "Let them go," but it didn't seem either of them was struggling or seeking to be let go. Rather, both seemed to want to be taken care of, be with their families. My Grandma Rees always said she wanted everything done to be kept alive as long as possible and she wanted to live with my mom when/if she could no longer live in her own house. My mother told the hospital, loudly, embarrassingly, the first time any doctor came into the Emergency Room where she was finally brought, short of breath, anemic, in kidney failure—in need of treatment, but… but my mother was quick to announce she was DNR or DNI—she would stumble over the words—and made it clear no resuscitation or life prolonging was desired. Apparently, her cemetery supplication to her grandparents had been heard: perhaps she thought they were coming for Leona.

Virginia Sue was my paternal grandmother. The last time I saw her and for most of the time I remember she had blond hair, dyed, with various grayish or whitish bits. The difference the last time was that the rest of her—skin, eyes, hospital gown—seemed the same gray-white-pale yellow shade. She seemed collapsed into her chair or into herself, struggled to see, but was still glad I was there, with Rockstar. She thanked me for the fruit I brought, berries maybe, and asked if I grew plums, someone had brought her lovely plums. Her husband, my grandfather, worked a farm for the church, in Lehi, mostly alfalfa. She had a small garden by the house, marigolds, maybe a tomato plant or two. She did have a few fruit trees, peach, plum, and made jam as well, I think, plum I do remember.

She petted Rockstar. He was with me the last time I visited my Grandma Rees at her care center as well. And now we visit their graves, leaving shells, Jordan almonds, stollen, occasionally flowers. The thing is though, I didn't have to bring anything or do anything, my grandmothers were always glad to see me, just to have me there.

I don't know. I was not in any position legally, physically, logistically, or morally to suggest that their lives may still have been meaningful and enjoyable, and then to offer to take care of them. And I have only my perspective, which may be wrong. Though, as Dr. Hardy says, "There is no capital 'T' Truth." What I know, I guess, is that I had two grandmothers who loved me and loved having me near them, something that seems so rare, nothing expected of me. And I loved them. And now I have no grandmothers. Because others, humans, God, fates, decided it was time for them to die.

I think how lucky I am still, when I sit with patients—refugees from Afghanistan, Somalia, Lithuania, Sudan—completely uprooted from homeland, alone, or nearly so.

Yesterday in clinic, I saw my first two afternoon patients as I returned from walking Rockstar during my lunch break. Iraqi refugees, they were sitting in the same general area of the waiting room, not together, both middle-aged women in layers of black, gold, dark blue fabrics. One 40 minutes early, one ten minutes early. Our interpreter had not yet arrived. After leaving Rock in my office with fresh water, I took my container of blueberries out to the waiting room and sat with them. I was never sure of the current pandemic protocols, but there was no one else in the waiting room and I offered each of them some blueberries, and both accepted. I don't speak Arabic. I sat diagonal from each of them, the three of us making a triangle, slipping blueberries under our face masks, chewing, smiling with our eyes.

When the interpretor arrived and we started her appointment, I asked the first woman, Entesar, through the interpreter, if she liked the blueberries. Entesar said they were interesting and fine and thanked me. And that she would never have thought to buy them, but has seen them, in the store. I touted their anti-inflammatory properties, Phyto nutrition, fiber, vitamins. And admitted they can be expensive, but frozen are equally nutritious, could be put on yogurt or salads.

Then I said. "They are my favorite."

Which, of course, was not medically relevant in the least. And added, equally needlessly, "What is your favorite?"

"Favorite fruit?" the interpreter and patient clarified.

"Yes."

Entesar said something and the interpreter did not know the English word. She said it was sort of like a peach only smaller, or at least not fuzzy.

"Apricot?" I offered.

Neither of them thought this was correct. The interpreter Googled and found a picture but not a word in English, for some reason. I now think it may have been a persimmon. I have not eaten one.

I think of these women. In a foreign land, far from the trees bearing their favorite fruits. Sitting in a clinic, passing through a pandemic with me, their doctor, and the small, though growing, community of other refugees. Uprooted, their eyes both restless and tired, an ocean away from family, from a homeland also in perpetual unrest.

Another patient of mine, Asmaan, went home to Afghanistan for the first time in 20 years. She had to wait for citizenship, for her PTSD and anxiety to be adequately controlled and then, finally, for a pandemic to be adequately controlled. She is, as far as I know, still there. She was delighted to be going. Scared, but so excited, her eyes lit in a way I had never seen. I think she will return, to Utah, her children ranging from toddler to 20 years old, the oldest and youngest both daughters, I think she would not leave them. But how it must be to go home. To see her mother, her aunts, her cousins. Her father was killed by the Taliban. I don't know how or why, and don't ask, unsure if that is to spare her or spare myself.

And back to Virginia Sue Johnson, my father's mother. Her family pedigree was indeed impressive. I wanted to be rooted, to know where I fit, maybe someday make a pilgrimage, seeking to see the lands of my ancestors. One day after finishing with patients in clinic, when I should have begun my report to Dragon, instead I went to FamilySearch.org and created a free account. I put in my name, I see myself as a rectangle on a chart, a family tree: Melissa Jean Bentley, female, in Salt Lake City, UT, alive. To my right, a line connects rectangle-me to a rectangles containing my parents. Their rectangle is thicker, they are both in it, a couple, though they divorced when I was eight and my mom has re-married. Then I follow the lines to the right of their rectangle which lead to their parents, my grandparents, and then lines from those rectangles lead to their parents and so on. If I click on the name in a rectangle, I can see "Life Events" and "Memories." Life Events are marriage, children and death. I suppose those are the only record-worthy life events—and since I have yet to manage any of these, I have none. An uneventful life. Surprisingly, given her six mostly active temple-going Mormon children (my dad being the exception), Virginia Sue Johnson Bentley's status is still listed as Living. I would have thought they might sign in regularly—but I have no idea. So, I add her Life Event of death, on Halloween, the year and location. It feels somehow wrong, as though I am too low down in the hierarchy of relations to do something so momentous, or as though I am changing her from living to dead by virtue of having updated the record. But what a record it is! Someone or ones in her family have been doing their gardening or genealogy or research or whatever it is, and the family tree or pedigree has been traced all the way back to the 5th Century, 400's A.D.! Rectangles and names and lines; some of them have "Memories" which might be a photo, or a land deed, or sometimes a lovely bit of a story.

But, I am still a godmother. And trying to be a good one, not an Air Fairy godmother. April turned five and six and seven during the pandemic. The Botanical Gardens were closed for a while, then opened on a timed entry basis, with masks to be worn indoors and anytime within view of anyone else outdoors, then just open again. We went to the Spring Plant Sale. I had a cartful of perennials, whose names I had learned and forgotten and relearned maybe 101 times in class. I let April choose something to take to her house to plant there.

I didn't always seek gardens or do gardening, though now I most certainly do. I remember when I was seven, my parents had separated, and my mother purchased the home where she lives now. It had what seemed an enormous back yard with a half-circle garden separating patio from lawn. It seemed so large, which might have been lovely, a large garden, but all she wanted planted then was petunias, an annual, so planted every year. We, her children who were so lucky to get to live there, had been assigned chores including yard work. First was weeding. My brother and sister and I each were responsible for a roughly equal section of the garden. The ground was hard, the weeds tenacious, the tools teaspoons. We had no trowel or shovel, each of us was allowed to use a spoon from the kitchen drawer, and our hands. We watered to try to soften the ground, dug and pulled, learned that getting the weeds out by the roots would keep them away longer—a bit of wisdom, my mother said, we could use in life. Then planting petunias, she would buy flat after flat, and would drop them in the garden, then we were to follow after, dig a hole with our spoon, plant each flower, then keep them watered and weeded through the spring and summer months, or as long as they lived. My mother noticed other yards in which the petunias covered the whole garden, no visible ground between each flower. She wondered why ours did not "fill-in" so nicely. I felt it was somehow my fault. I got some Miracle-Gro, not knowing at the time about the myriad harms of fertilizers. My section of flowers then had blue-green leaves—but didn't seem any more flowerful.

April chose a yellow Columbine, with its intricate yellow flowers in full bloom. I was surprised.

"Are you surprised?" she asked.

Sometimes children are frighteningly perceptive.

"I am," I said. "I thought you might choose a pink Bleeding Heart." Those have seemed to be her favorite in my back yard.

"Pink is not my favorite color anymore," she said. "Do you know what is?"

"Yellow," I said.

"How did you know?" she asked, seeming disappointed.

I stared at her Columbine.

She laughed and poked my arm.

"I still like pink too though, in case you got me something pink."

I did not have anything pink for her. She spends a fair bit of time with my dad and her mother's parents, and typically comes away with a pile of new items after each grandparent "sleep-over."

"Grampy got me pink gloves and a pink shovel and small sort of rake, but small, and I can still use them to plant this…" She looked up at me

"Columbine," I offered. One of 101 Plants to know.

"Columbine," she agreed. "I can still use them, even though pink is not my favorite color."

"Sure, of course you can," I said. "Or you could use a teaspoon, if the ground's not too hard."

Preserves

Still a child, I'm invited to watch, a privilege, the labors of my hero mother, the bloody crowning,

first a half-brother, later a half-sister.

Later still with my sister.

By then I, a half-doctor, or a bit more—invited nearer the birth bed, to stand between the shining thighs.

My sister struggles and shouts for a shot, and it stops—the pain and her pushing. I swim laps while she sleeps, pager nearby.

Crawl out like the Gollum, get dressed wet, back in time.

Her face saintly and sweaty, her son's head, shoulders, spine—he is warm, fine in my hands, I am swim-cool and still.

My white coat still sharp, my holding him wrong, the child's not mine.

Arms outstretch: my mother's, his, his father's, his nurse—

I ghostify. Slip unseen through the walls, slide along halls, along time.

They make children and grandchildren, new houses and vows.

A long time, a far shore. A past. Not a part. Apart.

A long walk on cliffs. It is fall. In this place, I belong. Only not.

Drawn to rocks, sea glass, shells. The smell of the sea, then repelled by the rot.

A sea pup, perhaps, beneath sea flies and beetles, surrounded by vultures. The sun warm and then hot.

The breeze now a gale.

All past, my past, mulled, pickled, preserved. Seen under glass, through the pale lemon shore-light.

Clarified or maligned? Magnified or distorted?

Weathered or warped?

Flotsam, fairy dust, foam…

My grandmothers passed. One the first of June, One Halloween night.

Forty-eight ribs caging two dear hearts caved-in;

sixteen cervical vertebrae hummocked.

Kidneys fill with stones. Pelvic bones break.

Hands become talons.

A better person might think of birds, wings, angels—

I do not.

I fish out two pairs of hands, free them from the sheet-shrouds.

Six fierce eyes fill with fluid.

Hands held fast.

The Forgetting and the Forgot.

I remember their shelves, heavy with bottles, peaches and pears.

Second freezers full of red jam and white frost.

Where have they gone? (repelled by the rot…)

I belong. Only not. I forget I am foreign, and the season and tides.

A sneaker wave, huge and heavy, hurls me over, brings me down.

Wholly drowned, no not quite, my own sneakers pulled off, I can
bob for a breath, for my bearing, then bear hard

East toward shore.

My nails scrape, toes claw. In swimsuit-sackcloth, I shiver ashore.

Sand is scalding, but I'm cold, and scared. Out of breath.

Hugging hard rocks, I sleep, held by stones.

Topcoat

"Wake up," I command.

Today, I do not visualize my mythical beast, yawning fire, reluctantly arising. My mind is too wiry, charged, not exactly sparking Dragon-ish, but linear, efficient. The nanosecond it takes for the microphone to turn green and vertical tries my patience. It happens rarely, but on occasion I long for a straightforward "normal" clinic practice. A urinary tract infection. A sore throat that is not a deadly virus. High blood pressure that is well managed on one medication, low sodium diet, daily exercise, and just needing medication refilled. Ailments that can be cured, or clearly treated, understood; cases clicked through, out in time for a walk with Rockstar.

"Opal is a 60 year-old woman with chronic heart and lung disease, obesity, other conditions here with chief complaint of dyspnea." I erase dyspnea. "I can't get my breath." Something learned in medical school, residency, and which I perpetually forget, or let slip—chief complaint is the patient's chief complaint. Very few of my patients, if any, would complain of dyspnea.

"She reports that she has been sick for a month, during which she at some point did a home COVID test which she thinks was negative. She missed her pulmonary and cardiology appointments, and rescheduled with the pulmonologist but went to the wrong office and was too sick and too late to go to the correct location. She notes that she has gained weight and thinks she might be retaining water. On questioning, she thinks she did take the new medicine, it started with an F maybe (an SGLT2 inhibitor, for her heart, blood sugar, kidneys) and she didn't notice any problem with it but doesn't remember to take pills in the evening and thought that she was supposed to take it in the morning. She doesn't feel that her inhaler is working and wants to try a different one but not one that would cause a yeast infection in her mouth. She notes that she has difficulty with stooling at night in bed and that in the past she had a problem with her intestine, she thinks it was a mega colon, and had to have surgery and has been sort of okay but now worse and wonders if there is something she can take for that. She notes that she visited her sister, Jade." (Jade is also my patient, a woman who struggles with methamphetamine abuse/addiction, but also with obesity—hypo-ventilation syndrome—about 150 pounds overweight, she is, literally, suffocating under her own body mass; not common in meth users, in my experience; but my patients are, after all, extraordinary.)

"Patient reports that she tried using her sister's oxygen for a while and felt better…"

I go on, then fall back on a custom command "The interested reader," which will input "The interested reader is referred to prior notes for complete history and other information."

What did I do before Dragon? I look at my hands, now spared the hours of typing. It is winter, and three fingertips on the right and one on the left are split open. I do not have enough body fat to stay warm, or I wash and/or alcohol them too much, or I fear it is a waste of time to get mittens I forgot going out the door. My fault if I am not tough enough, am forgetful. I have super-glued them, but need to again, there is blood on my white coat, I notice. They hurt.

My wiry brain seems to wander for a moment, I check my email and see an advertisement from the local nail salon. Some time ago, my aunt in California, Lura, sent a gift card. It is a building a few blocks from my home, and I walked there, in the pandemic, after ensuring their infection control protocols, and their use of organic, vegan, cruelty-free products. They have sent an email, the salon, Top Coat. I should unsubscribe or mark as junk and phishing. Instead, I click the link and book a hand treatment for the end of the day... and then pick up my dictation thread.

In social history, I relate, "Patient works as a cleaner, and notes that she has had difficulty taking time off work for appointments. However, she has been too sick to work the last month, as noted above, and is very worried about finances. She has cut back smoking to a pack every three days."

I say, "Smoking Cessation," and Dragon reveals to all, but in particular to billing, that I spent over 5 minutes discussing harmful effects of tobacco use, detailed these effects, and detailed the ways I described that I could help, including patches, gum…

Opal is too ill to come in to see me or to keep the specialist appointments—too sick to work and so without an income. And yet—and now I want to weep—she has brought me a gift. I have not opened it. I will put it under my tree at home. I have an artificial tree, pre-lit, a decade or so old, undecorated, tall and slim. I do open her card. It wishes me a Merry Christmas and Happy New Year and thanks me for "everything you do for me, you make me want to live when I was ready to give up! You're the best…"

Oh, Opal, if only that were true—if only I could fix your heart and lungs and bowels and abusive son and bad back and bad credit from a bad husband with drugs and debt and…

Instead, here is how the visit with Opal went. I knock on the door, wash my hands, greet her. I go over medications, do a nebulizer treatment in clinic, which helps. "It's as though the lights are turned on again!" she says. So, I get a nebulizer and vials of medication for her to use at home. I let her choose which inhaler of two that are, in essence, equivalent, looks better to her. I have them on a picture in my exam rooms, commonly prescribed inhalers, mostly so that when patients describe what they need, or don't like, based upon the shape or color of the device, I have some hope of figuring it out. I check her oxygen levels walking, an MA holding her elbow, a pulse oximeter on her finger as they make laps around the clinic. And then I arrange to check her oxygen overnight as well, so she doesn't have to use Jade's oxygen: Jade should be using it herself. At rest, she doesn't qualify for oxygen, according to Medicaid requirements; her saturation level is above 90%. If she answers the phone when the home oxygen testing company contacts her and if she can manage to pick up the overnight testing device and if she wears it and it doesn't fall off and returns it to the company and if they report the data and email or fax it to my MA, I will have this information. Many ifs, many of which often fall through…

I suggest things for her bowels, preferring not to do another referral, to colorectal surgery or gastroenterology, as she is struggling to get to the heart and lung appointments— which we reschedule. I do labs to check her chronic kidney failure, blood sugar, anemia severity. I tell her that her newly dyed pink hair is smashing. It is a bit gorgeous. I wish her a Merry Christmas, and put her on my schedule in one week, hoping that by having her back quickly, she will not get worse, will not be too sick to come, will not have stopped any medications, will be able to go over labs with me and maybe a half hour will be enough time.

This, or some summary of it is what I tell Dragon, noting for the billers, or maybe for myself, that I have taken 70 minutes for Opal's appointment today. For myself so that when someone asks about work and I say it was a busy day and they ask how many patients I saw and it is nothing like the 30-35 patient encounters their family practice clinician schedules routinely—so that I can somehow try to justify myself, that I am not lazy, Air Fairy, am thorough, am careful. Maybe.

I tell my medical assistants that I will need to leave as soon as I am done seeing our last patient, for an appointment. I do not tell them it is at Topcoat. I am secretly ashamed. But I have booked it, too late to cancel, have to do it now to get the deal they sent in the email, I rationalize. I make it there five minutes late, and apologize. It seems okay, the nail artist is finishing her break, the very pregnant supervisor takes me to a chair, and hands me a menu, Would I like something to eat or drink? I am masked, of course, and the nail artist assigned to me, seeing this, masks as well, which I appreciate. I hesitate with the menu, I am thirsty, but it seems unsanitary. I trust myself to dispense blueberries to my patients, pass out citrus fruit, but I have to be cautious, I can't trust the salon and can't risk being sick and unable to work myself. The chair in which I will sit is too low-down and too soft and the back lies back too far. It can do many massage actions, can heat up, can be completely horizontal, but it seems it cannot become just a normal, straight-backed chair. I don't like it, it seems to swallow me, and I can't feel the edges of myself, somehow. It is, however, quite distanced from any others, and is by a window. I say, throwing out caution, "I would love a Diet Coke, thank you," and imagine Dr. Hardly throttling me. Diet Coke—useless, no nutritive value, bad for bones which are already osteoporotic, bad for teeth which break and cost a fortune to maintain, years of poor diet. Ensure is not on the menu, however. I could have just had water. But I wanted to—what?—enjoy something, be frivolous for a moment? It's wrong, the guilt outweighs any pleasure.

"Okay, anything to eat? I recommend the orange garble garble garble," she replies.

I have no idea what she said and mumble nothing in reply, just make my usual humming noise, I guess. It must sound like an affirmative, however, as she brings me a small chocolate candy with a picture of an orange on the package, along with the diet soda.

My nail artist is named Celine. She has amazing 1.5-inch-long nails, mostly hot pink with gray lines—what I would call "crazy paving" or "ground glass" appearance—something that is used to describe the appearance of a particular group of lung diseases on radiologic studies. But her thumbs are lime green; thumbnails, I mean. She puts on purple plastic gloves, and immediately the nails spike through. It is fascinating.

I used to not talk, to strangers, clerks at the store, nail artists. I think of myself as a private person, maybe introverted, maybe shy, maybe distrustful. When I was younger, I remember going places with my grandmother, who was a wonderful talker. She was sure to let the saleswoman know that we were out shopping for my birthday, informing the grocery bagger that I am spending the night with her, that I am her granddaughter, and she is letting me have my choice for dinner. I often chose to eat cottage cheese with pineapple, I loved how she put one large leaf of iceberg lettuce on a small plate, then a round mound of cottage cheese, a pineapple ring, and a maraschino cherry perfectly centered on top.

I think of those moments, not momentous. Just days, small exchanges. I have heard people with children and spouses say that the happiest moments of their lives were their wedding day, or the birth of a child. That they didn't know how to love until then. Once, I asked Dr. Hardy about this, Was your happiest moment when you got married, or when you became a father, did you not know how to love until you had a child?

He said those moments are memorable, I think, but that happy moments are not the huge life pinnacle events. It is the store clerk who always has a joke for him. What a gift it is, that joke, that connection. It is watching his dogs take off through the snow at the old golf course, lightning fast, pure joy.

It is a gift to be here, to meet Celine. I still do not share things about myself, in general, it's too strange that I am a doctor and have no significant other, no children, in Utah, at my age… The culture, mostly Mormons, encourages early marriage and large families, and for mothers to stay home to care for their children. But I love hearing about—well, stories—and although I love my work, utterly, in these circumstances, I can listen differently, no diagnosis, no treatment. A gift.

And Celine is from Tijuana, the one city in Mexico to which I have been. Long ago, when it was possible to easily walk across the border from California. I ask, How was it there?

And she tells me. She lived in a small house with three sisters and one brother and her grandmother and her parents. They ate tacos for breakfast lunch and dinner, and she loved them. Sometimes marinated goat meat, sometimes carne asada, sometimes beans. Her grandmother had a dog, Louisa, who had puppies, including one Celine acquired and has now.

Then, I do tell her about Rockstar, of course, show her the lock screen on my phone, a photo of Rockstar, his deep brown eyes and dark lashes and brows. And she tells me about her dogs, she has two now. Looney weighs twelve pounds and always wants to have a ball, plays for hours.

Fortunately/unfortunately, Celine's husband was not working outside the home, with "la pandemia," and so has been home to do endless ball with Looney. Her other dog, Pan-chan, weighs five pounds. Pan-chan was acquired from a neighbor for whom she had been an emotional support animal. When the neighbor got COVID and had to go to the hospital, Celine and her husband agreed to look after his dog. She offered to send him a photo, and did, but he did not reply. He died. So Pan Chan, whose dark black hair has probably 12 little bows in all the pictures I am shown, has stayed with them. And Celine thinks this dog has been an emotional support for her husband, who is doing what work he can from home.

And she talks and I listen and watch, and for a moment, the moment is lovely. Celine's purple-gloved hands with pink and green nail spikes put cold mud, then warm towels, then cream on my cracked red ones. She has a "fill-in-the-cracks" magic cream, that may not be as durable as super-glue, but feels good for the moment. I have almost no fingernails, they don't grow, just sort of peel off, but she files and buffs gamely, applies a vegan, cruelty-free, organic polish, which I have chosen for the name as much as the shade: Inner beauty. It is a wintry blue-silver.

Then I look at my watch. So much time has passed, I have not been careful, I have not been paying attention, so selfish, so careless. All this time, not working, not studying, not checking for any messages or doing anything at all useful. Sitting way too long. I have to stand up, keep trying to leave as she says, No, "drying drops" next, no, wait longer to dry, do you want to lie back and have massage from chair? NO! I have wasted so much time already, what was I thinking! No, thanks, I say, I better go, Rockstar is waiting…

This she seems to accept, and I leave, tipping ridiculously, but Looney's balls, and Pan Chan's bows and her husband struggling to work—it all is a good cause, a good use of a few extra dollars, I think.

And why have I been here, luxuriating, looking at fingernails, sitting in a too-soft chair, drinking soda, when my patient, Opal, struggles to breathe, cleans apartments, has an infinitely complicated life, it seems? (Though, I recall, she does have startlingly long fake fingernails.) And why did I feel the need to escape, not revealing myself as a doctor, just a dog lover, to listen to Celine, to connect, but in a way that surely doesn't matter? Not healing, not curing, not preventing illness. There is a pandemic. I had my nails done and drank a Diet Coke. What was I thinking? Not thinking, perhaps, a slip, a chance to learn, to do better, to stay focused next time, on my work, my patients, not myself. On bodies and insides, hearts and souls, not outside appearance, fingernails, hair bows.

Cold

I am cold. It is cold, but I am being a wimp with the cold, shivering, not being tough. For Christmas, as a gift, our gymnastic coaches gave each of us a voucher for the human performance lab at the University, to do metabolic and body composition testing. So, I am wearing only my swimsuit and a tight-fitting cap. I step onto a scale, weight is recorded, and then I climb into what looks like a small space capsule. According to the lab brochure, the Bod Pod machine I am about to enter uses "air displacement plethysmography" to determine the relative amounts of lean and fat mass comprising myself. Or my body. I have only to hold still and breath normally. Jim, the older physiologist who runs the campus lab, starts the machine. They do the test twice. Usually. He does it again. Then again.

When I am out and dressed, he shows me my results, and the reason for the repeats. The printout shows that for a woman:

Risky (high body fat)	>40%
Excess Fat	30.1—40%
Moderately Lean	22.1—30%
Lean	18.1—22%
Ultra Lean	15—18%
Risky (low body fat)	<15%

My result is 1.8%. Which does not seem possible. Is not. I study medicine. Fat is essential to support organs, to form bone marrow, to coat nerves to—to just be a body—to not freeze. My coaches seem impressed but slightly nervous or confused, then opt for the celebratory, praise, impressed stance. Jim says, "If you were my daughter, I would be worried." I do not know what to say. I say, "Sorry."

So, since I am not your daughter, you are not worried? Or I have done something wrong, but it's okay since I am not your daughter? Or someone should be worried, but you, Jim, are not? Where do I fit in the family of things?

My therapist and dietitian are worried. "What would you tell a patient with that result? If you were your patient what would you do?"

But it is another impossible question. I am not my patient. So, I have no idea, since it isn't a possibility. I never will be my patient, and I am different somehow, Air Fairy reminds me: yes, people need body fat, but I don't, clearly, because I am okay, just need to be tough.

On call nights, overnight in-hospital call, usually around 8:30 or 9:00 I start to get especially cold, my body still thinking that it is time for sleep, the normal cellular, hormonal process still untrained, the body clock not quite shut off. The pull towards the blanket seems almost magnetic, just wrap in a warm blanket for a few moments, then get back to typing notes, reviewing lab results on the computer, studying patients and their diseases. Fortunately, I am saved from the seduction of sleep, when I might miss something: my pager goes off. It is the well-known ER number. A patient to admit. I head down the stairs to meet her. I wonder if a storm is coming, my foot is aching where it was broken. "Things are strongest where they are broken," comes to mind—did I read that in a textbook, or a novel? Or a poem? I speak "The Wild Geese," Mary Oliver, under my breath, glad to have it by heart.

You do not have to be good.
You do not have to walk on your knees
for a hundred miles through the desert repenting.
You only have to let the soft animal of your body
    love what it loves.
Tell me about despair, yours, and I will tell you mine.
  Meanwhile the world goes on.
Meanwhile the sun and the clear pebbles of the rain
 are moving across the landscapes,
 over the prairies and the deep trees,
 the mountains and the rivers.
Meanwhile the wild geese, high in the clean blue air,
   are heading home again.
Whoever you are, no matter how lonely,
the world offers itself to your imagination,
calls to you like the wild geese, harsh and exciting
 over and over announcing your place
    in the family of things.

"Tell me of your despair," I say to the patient as I enter her cubicle in the ER. Though perhaps not so poetically. For that is your job, my patient, tell me your despair. And I will not tell you mine, my despair. For that is my job, to be your doctor.

Some questions I might ask Ms. Oliver: "What if I very much want to be good? Not have to, but want to? What if not being good, at medicine, means that a patient is harmed, or dies? What if a soft self sleeps and misses a crucial call, or a critical piece of information is missed, and my sleeping is the cause of another's suffering? What if my animal self loves to flip and fly and run and loves to help patients feel better, to learn and know what to do and to do it—but in the process of that, there is no softness, and if there is: fragility, fractures?

Maybe just one question for Mr. Nietzsche: What if in the process of trying to grow stronger I am also dying, not all at once, but by degrees: 180-degree split leap, 360-degree full twist back flip; medical doctor, M.D.

Faith Healing

Power is out on the mountain. *The whole mountain is experiencing an outage. We have no estimate for restoration at this time. Why not visit the Lookout for a warm hot chocolate and pastry?*

Ivy, who I think is an AI being, but am not quite sure, has texted me this information.

Crews are available, the resort's next text message reads. *Would you like a blanket or flashlight?*

Yes, yes, both, I am freezing and I hate having no power, I text back.

Then I worry this will gum up the system, only YES /NO/ STOP is allowed—and I just put, *YES.*

It is the second Christmas of the pandemic, and I am staying in a Sundance Resort Mandan cabin. There is a group of perhaps a dozen two-story "cabins" spread out along the Provo River. I am surrounded by aspen, maple, spruce, and oak trees, so that in the summer it feels almost as if I am in a luxurious tree house, green leaves shining through open windows; and the balcony overhangs the river, so near that the sound of the river drowns all other noise. I cannot hear peoples' voices or the sound of traffic; and occasionally I can't even hear Air Fairy. When I first came here it was June, five years ago, before the pandemic, and my grandmother had just died. I hiked to a waterfall, did pottery, made soap using local wildflowers and organic fats; I visited horse stables, I shouted at and ran away from a moose. I listened to moving water, painted with watercolor, drew with pastels, got entirely messy doing each of these and felt, finally, that I could breathe. That first visit, I could not bear the fact of my grandma dead. I felt then that whatever faith I thought I had in heaven, of somehow seeing my grandmother again, was false. Or at least untested, utterly weak.

I have visited multiple times since then, when able to take some days from work. Work that I love but... worry about my patients, the chaos of the inner-city clinic for the underserved, my inability to know all I felt I needed to "do no harm," to help. I feel deeply responsible for those in my care, for whom I care enormously, but at times I feel without the resources necessary. And am physically, mentally, morally depleted. Work with the poor, traumatized, chronically—and—complicatedly-ill patients is never easy. But all stresses were infinitely deepened while practicing in the pandemic. So, a respite: here was space, beauty and wildness. Rockstar was welcome to accompany me everywhere, and did, getting equally muddy, clay-y, paint-y…

Most of my visits have been in the "off-season," not in the winter, when it is more expensive—it is largely known as a ski resort. The resort was built and the land was preserved by the actor Robert Redford, also known for the Sundance Film Festival he created. I tell myself that staying here is supporting nature conservation and the arts, which is true. The glass is all recycled, the native peoples who first lived here are named, thanked. I also asked about a discounted rate, since I am a local and, I told them, shamefully (how can I be exhausted when so privileged, able—unlike my patients, and so many who are sick—to escape?) a doctor exhausted by the pandemic. But it is true—sick patients, fear and grief, and also a society tired of a virus that persists and people who seem less and less willing to mask, to isolate. Sundance seemed, again, a place to breathe, I have my own cabin and so should be safe, not spreading virus, but maybe not quite so alone. Even if Rockstar and I are alone in our cabin, we can venture out to the art studio, we can pass bundles of bright hats, goggles, ski pants, knowing there are people inside. Rock can shamelessly exchange rear-end sniffs with other dogs. And yet. How is it fair for me to come here? My patients—in small, multi-family apartments, in the shelter next to the clinic, on the reservation with intermittent power outages and some without indoor water. It's not right. And I am here anyway. And I can breathe. And prepare to re-enter clinic work, better for the holiday. I hope.

I am no great downhill skier, preferring to put on my 50+ year-old wooden skis, with my tennis shoes, to head out with Rockstar to a park, golf course, foothill trail. There is no waiting and freezing in line or on lifts, no pass that costs quadruple the price of my yard sale skis, no falling hard down the slope—only soft falls, mostly level ground, with the cross-country workout keeping me toasty. Usually. During this stay, though, the weather has shown its ultimate power. After last winter, the first pandemic winter, we all became accustomed to outdoor-only visits—the way I could keep some contact with my goddaughter. Then there was a freak windstorm that uprooted enormous trees, followed by a cold snap last fall. It left me freezing and without power for three days. Now, I fancied myself prepared, utterly, for any weather conditions. Better than any Boy Scout. REI did curbside service, I bought just about everything warm, solar or battery powered, waterproof, and/or light-producing that they had in stock.

And besides, I have grown up near the Utah mountains and have spent time in upper Michigan and Quebec—I am no stranger to snow. But here at Sundance, I have been beaten. The trick was rain in the middle of snow. With a 39" base, it then rained and then again snowed. And then snowed more. And my snowshoes or skis sank through the powder into the 8" of slush-ice water underneath. My spikes kept me from sliding—but there was nothing to keep me from sinking. My First People boots from Canada were waterproof and warm to a point. But my legs grew exhausted. And even endlessly-energetic Rockstar, having to bound through mounds twice his height, wore out. Mushers Secret on his paws kept ice balls from forming but couldn't keep him out of the ice water either. The explosions for avalanche control terrified him. We were beaten.

More text messages from Ivy.

All lifts are closed. The Lookout is closed, but the Owl bar remains open, why not come in for company and drinks?

Warning: avalanche control measures anticipated. Be prepared for road closures and sound of explosives during this time.

You are slipping a bit, Ivy, I think, unkindly—we have already heard those explosives, without the pre-warning; though if she is not a real person, is it unkind? I suppose she is programmed by someone real, yes?

The Owl Bar is closed, Ivy texts.

Rockstar and I had ventured down to "base camp" where the harried boys at the front desk assured me I was on the list for blankets and flashlights. Though I had prepared to be out in the cold, I had assumed power in the cabin—for light, for re-charging all my battery-powered warmth, boiling my hand warmers to reset them, or just to rest—wimpily warming up for spells. We stop at a communal fire pit for a while, then I fear I will be too tired to make it back to our cabin. It is in truth probably less than half a mile to its door, but with the deep snow, this is a formidable distance—so we head up the hill. There are chest-high wooden posts with solar lights along the path leading up to the cabin, and though snow has reached the tops of the posts, it has not yet covered the lights. For a while, at least, I was not cold. But I knew this would not last, and I was scared—of the dark, the cold, my lack of faith—or fear of Air Fairy I guess, too—could I manage? I was exhausted. But still I could be aware that it was dazzlingly beautiful. Quiet, white. There was movement, snowflakes falling in seeming perpetuity, and yet somehow also utterly still.

Still, Still, Still, I thought, humming the winter song in lieu of my llama-hum-strange-anxious noise.

For a panicked moment I am not sure if I have keys, but I do. I smile at the key chain. It was made for me, of leather and metal, by a patient, Yezen. A man from Iraq, whom the medical assistants find scary. I confess that I also feel a bit intimidated by him, at times. He has a loud, low voice, and expressive dark eyes with thick brows and lashes. He has something very wrong with the anatomy of his sinuses or ear canals, or both, having been injured in an explosion. Last time he came to see me, he refused to return to see otolaryngology—ENTs. I have referred him to two, he has seen two, not liking the first, then feeling the second was not helpful either. The interpreter has told me that the drops and pills I gave him worked—but now they are not working. But he feels I know better than the specialists and he, Yezen, will do what I advise, but he needs new medicines now.

I am torn. I fear that Yezen has said that "I know better than the specialists" to flatter me so that I will keep ordering things and not insist that he return to ENT. Often, with patients, I am well aware that as an internist, a doctor for adults, usually adults with multiple complicated chronic conditions, I do not have the training that a specialist does, for a particular condition. Cardiologists are needed for my patients with severe coronary disease, valve or heart failure; neurologists for patients with uncontrolled epilepsy; nephrologists for patients with kidney failure in need of dialysis; and so on. And yet— I also know that at my clinic I am blessed with, usually, time—to listen to patients, to see them again and again and again, to hear their stories, meet their families, see how they respond to treatments. We receive funding through the IHS, through Medicaid and Medicare and—honestly I don't know exactly—but I don't have to meet certain requirements for number of patients in a day, I have only a salary, no "incentive" pay based on RVUs—relative value units. I have time for each patient's appointment.

And also, I have time—over weeks and months and years with patients—to come to know and, though I fear it is somehow wrong to say, time to truly love them. And time to read, research, think about conditions and symptoms, treatment options. The pandemic has added a tangle to my thought thread—patients now are afraid to go the hospital, seeing wards of COVID patients on the news. And I am aware of hospitals at or over capacity, and of specialists, especially those who care for the critically ill, being overworked, exhausted mentally and physically.

And yet… I cannot look into Yezen's nasal passage to frontal sinus, or ear canals in the same way that and otolaryngologist can, and I cannot surgically correct pathologic blockages, or see and drain collected infection, abscesses that could cause destruction or lead to bacteremia, brain infection, permanent damage, death. Yezen is diabetic, putting him at risk for mucor, mucormycosis, a particularly destructive fungal infection of the sinuses.

At his last visit, he added another knot to the tangle. I walked into the exam room, washing my hands, then as I turned to face him, he pulled out this black leather key chain, with red border stitching and my name in silver: Melissa on one side and Bentley on the other. He had made it. I was amazed, both at his having this skill, and that he would make this for me. I thought to refuse it, but also realized probably no one else could use a key chain with my name on it—and I would be uncomfortable if someone did. And, he smiled. Had I seen him smile before? Rarely; maybe never. I smiled.

"Shukran," I said.

An even bigger smile. Is it possible? This was Yezen—but yes.

"Afwan," he replied.

Then, through the interpreter, he tells me, again, that the last ENT did not help, and he knows that I can order something that will cure his ear pain, he just cannot tolerate it any longer.

I take a deep breath. I look in his ear again. The passage is clogged with wax, debris, and, I fear, infectious discharge. He has no fever. I will do a CBC to be sure his white blood count is normal. I will treat with different drops, consider putting in a wick/draining, but fear doing damage. I will order oral antibiotics and anti-fungal pills. I will see him back very soon.

"He says he is very sure it will work, and that you are the best," the interpreter says. "He also wants a different shampoo for his dandruff."

I order a different shampoo, thank Yezen for the gift, tell him he must let me know if he is not better or any worse. Then I will insist that he see ENT—and that he could see dermatology for his scalp as well—?

And of course, I tell Dragon all of this, being very sure to document the multiple times that I advised seeing otolaryngology and that I detailed my concerns and risks—which I did. Not wanting to scare Yezen, but needing to be sure he understood, was aware.

And should I tell Dragon of the gift? And did the gift make me more willing to think harder, to come up with a different medication to try?

And does Yezen's belief that I can cure or at least treat, help him—how much might that actually help? Certainly, studies show the placebo effect is powerful.

And what studies have been done regarding the doctor's faith? If I believe what I am doing will help, or if I believe in a God who will help me help my patients, keep me from doing harm, heal them—does that add anything to my treatment plan, augment my best medicine guess? And if I am plagued by doubt, self-doubt or God-doubt—does that make treatment success less likely, pills less powerful?

I think of two poems by favorite poets.

"Some Questions You Might Ask, Mary Oliver," I think.

Is the soul solid, like iron? Or is it tender and breakable, like the wings of a moth in the beak of the owl?

Who has it, and who doesn't?

I keep looking around me. The face of the moose is as sad as the face of Jesus.

The swan opens her white wings slowly.

In the fall, the black bear carries leaves into the darkness...

And so on. Dr. Hardy and I discuss Mary Oliver as MO, we trade poems. Also, we love David Whyte.

I want to write a poem about Faith, David Whyte, I think.

I want to write about faith, about the way the moon rises over cold snow, night after night, faithful even as it fades from fullness, slowly becoming that last curving and impossible sliver of light before the final darkness.

But I have no faith myself,

I refuse it the smallest entry...

As I take out my keys, I bless Dr. Hardy, who suggested I wear a small fanny-pack, in which I keep a tiny case with ID and cards, cell phone, and keys. Always so compulsive in care of patients, in cleaning, in so many ways, when I am especially stressed, I lose them, leave them places—key, wallet, phone... So his suggestion.

Rockstar and I go into the cabin. No power. My phone battery is at 17%.

Ivy texts me, *Crews are out, we have flashlights and blankets, and the greatest snow on earth.*

I wonder who she is, or who added that cheery reminder. I wonder if I am on the list for blankets and flashlights and if the crews are out. I wonder if Yezen has gone deaf. I wonder if I should pray. I do, often, pray, or try. For patients, for Dr. Hardy, for myself to not do harm, to not miss things, to know what to do. "Can prayers be harmful?" I wonder at times. If I am doing it "incorrectly," or am undeserving of help, lacking faith. But I pray also for forgiveness, to deserve help, and I hope that the God to whom I try to pray is indeed more benevolent than Air Fairy—whom I still reliably try to serve.

Charlene

Charlene winced as she walked across the waiting room, limped across really, and I winced as I watched her: clearly she was in pain. I was rooming her myself—something my medical assistants usually do—because we were, again, short-staffed. Several medical assistants were out sick, with colds, the old "normal" type of coronavirus, not Covid-19. But we were never entirely sure of the accuracy of tests in those days, and patients, understandably, did not want to be in close contact with someone coughing, sneezing, sick. So I was collecting some patients myself, and I really didn't want Charlene, a patient at high-risk for infection, sitting in the waiting room any longer than absolutely necessary.

Both masked, of course, I smiled at her anyway, and saw the smile returned in her green eyes, despite the pain. I offered her my arm, she seemed hesitant, and I wished I looked sturdier, stronger to her. But at last she took my elbow, shoulder, and we made our way to the closest exam room.

"What hurts, what is wrong?" I asked, worried. Charlene had metastatic lung cancer, known spots of invasion included her liver and adrenal glands, but I feared it might have spread to her bones, and that she had a fracture. She has a bad hip, arthritis severe enough most orthopedists would have advised replacement, but usually she doesn't limp.

"I don't know Dr. B.," she said, "it's just, my leg is swollen, I've been elevating it, but it's still hot and swollen and hurts."

She sat heavily, seemed to sigh with relief. It was summer then, and she had on short pants, so I was easily able to see what she meant, the problem. Her left leg, from the calf down, was indeed swollen and red. Her left foot barely fit into her white sandals, the straps painfully tight cutting into the flesh of her foot, above her hot-pink toenails. I took off the shoe and examined her leg. There was a "palpable cord," as the textbook describes, a firm rope, probably her popliteal vein, the vein just behind the knee, but possibly extending up the thigh into her femoral vein. Both her cancer and the medication she took to treat it made her at high risk for deep venous thrombosis, or DVT, a blood clot within large veins. Clot in the palpable veins was probably blocking the normal flow of blood from her foot back up to her heart. Not only was this painful, it was dangerous, as the clot or portions of it could break off, travel back up the leg veins to the heart, and from there be pumped out into the lungs- a pulmonary embolism. This could be fatal if large enough, or if the patient's lungs were already compromised- as was certainly the case with Charlene.

An ultrasound quickly showed this to be the diagnosis. I explained to Charlene the diagnosis, the treatment, the serious nature, but I also wanted to be reassuring, it was good she had come in. Because of her cancer and the risks, I advised getting started on blood thinners in the hospital, where her blood pressure, heart and lungs could be monitored. She utterly refused.

"No, Doc. I'll take my chances. The hospitals are full of tired doctors and nurses and patients dying of Covid. No thanks. Just do the best you can for me, and that'll be just fine."

It was hard to argue with the part about the hospital. Again, I felt that pandemic despair, pressure, fear, impossibility. I did not have the expertise to do what was needed, the monitors, an IV heparin drip...And yet she wasn't wrong about our hospitals, in the middle of a Covid surge.

"Okay." I said. "I will give you a shot of a blood thinner, and then have you start taking pills that will keep you from developing more clot in your leg. They won't dissolve the clot, but with your blood thinned, your body will absorb the clot on its own over the next days and weeks. If you are not on blood thinners, the clot will grow, making the risks of a pulmonary embolism even higher."

"Perfect," Charlene said. "See, I knew you could take care of me."

"But," I said, "If you start feeling short of breath or have pain in your chest, you must go the hospital immediately. This could mean your clot went to your lungs, and you could die."

"Got it Doc, sure," she said.

I had no idea if she really would. But other than giving her compression stockings, crutches, a pulse oximeter to make sure her oxygen levels stayed in the 90s, in the normal range, and offering something for pain, there seemed little else I could do. She declined my offer to wheel her home in a wheelchair—she lived in the women's homeless shelter, next door to the clinic. Something that terrified me—a pandemic, a patient with COPD, chronic obstructive pulmonary disease, also called "emphysema," not to mention lung cancer, and on chemotherapy which weakened her immune system—living in such close quarters. I confess that, perhaps unfairly, I assumed that the shelter lacked good sanitation, cleanliness.

Charlene was the model patient, model citizen mid-pandemic. She was never unmasked. She carried a bottle of hand sanitizer with her, always, as well as a large tub of Clorox wipes, something the shelter kept in stock, and allowed her to do. On the rare occasions they were low on masks or sanitizer, she would get some from her oncologist's office, or from me. She traveled by bus every three weeks to the infusion center at the cancer hospital, about twenty miles to the south, for Opdivo, or "the diva" as Charlene called it, an IV immunotherapy. She also took Iressa, ("the I-pills"), an oral anti-cancer drug.

I could not help but think, as I watched her hobbling out, that it wasn't fair. That if a person has to have metastatic lung cancer, at least she should have a car, a home, a partner or children to help care for her. Not a homeless shelter, especially during a pandemic, a new virus that preferentially seemed to affect the lungs. Once I made the mistake of saying something — I'm so sorry you have to deal with all this, it seems unfair — something like that. She set me straight, by asking me if I knew the cost of her medicines — I did not, and said so — that I assumed they were pretty expensive. And that I feared this would become yet another trial, hardship.

"The diva is $7,787 each treatment," she said. "Not including the cost of the nausea medicine they give me or the snacks or the nurses' salaries, all of that. And the I-pills, just one a day, $8,325 a month, assuming the month has 30 days. And you know what? My Medicaid and Medicare cover them. I don't pay a cent. Can you imagine? You can't get luckier than that. Someone, God or the government or both, thinks that I'm worth that much. I can't believe it, but I'm grateful. I got no room to complain, none."

Like so many patients, she taught me, inspired me. Fortunately, her leg swelling improved, there was no sign that the clot had caused any catastrophe. Given her risks, cancer and at least one blood clot—the biggest risk for having another—we kept her on the "blood thinning" pills. They cost around $700 for a month's supply, small change. And Charlene didn't have to pay anything out of pocket. She seemed stable overall, continuing her rigorous practices to avoid getting Covid. She ate separated from anyone else at the shelter, by more than six feet, and until it got really cold—sometimes even then if it wasn't raining/snowing/blowing too hard, as she put it—she ate at the picnic tables in the courtyard. I saw her monthly through the fall.

When I saw her in December, I asked about her plans for the holiday, if the shelter had anything special planned.

"Sure, they always do something nice, but I won't be there," she said.

"Oh?"

"My friend got housing, Section 8, his turn, so some of us are getting together there for Christmas dinner," she said.

Before I could start with my advice she continued, "Don't worry, we will take all the precautions, he has bad lungs too and still smokes, we are using paper and plastic, we've walked out the six feet and set chairs there through the apartment, we will leave the balcony door open while we are there, and if they have tests at the shelter, we will all take a covid test before we get together, so of course if anyone has it they will be uninvited. Plus, it is just four of us, and we all do—well you know. Distance, masks, wipes."

"Well. Okay," I say. "Just please be so careful. What are you going to eat?" For some reason, though I eat very few things, it interests me to know what other people have, especially for special meals.

"Gio is making lasagna," she tells me. "It is, apparently, an old family recipe, something he got from his birth mother, whom he met just before she died. Gio was adopted, in New York City, his family was, of course, Italian. He was beaten by his adoptive father. One punch in the eye damaged him so badly that he actually lost it—the eye. He has a glass eye..."

As she is telling me this story, I realize I know him. He is my patient too. Giovanni, to me. And was homeless, staying at another shelter.

Among other things, he struggled with recurrent skin infections. His wife—a woman who out-weighed him five times over and pushed a tiny dog in a baby stroller into the exam room at his appointments, which she invariably attended—told me that the problem was that he refused to shower at the shelter. People were beaten up or abused in the showers, and so his skin got dirty, infested, she said. Of course I cannot tell Charlene that he is my patient, privacy rules—but I hope that he is the one who got the subsidized housing, that he has an apartment with a pristine shower, that he can take warm safe showers anytime he wants, then apply the cream I prescribe, thick as shortening, that his skin will heal, that somehow that will salve, soften, soothe deeper wounds.

Charlene tells me that Gio has been saving up, using part of his "food stamps" for months to get the ingredients for the lasagna, garlic bread, and layer cake he insists on providing. She says they offered to go in, but he declined. It was his gift. He did say he doesn't care for any green stuff, so if anyone wants salad, they're on their own to provide, he won't touch the stuff. My nutritional counseling must need work.

There is a city- or state- or nation-wide shortage of toilet paper, for reasons that are not clear. Something to do with shipping or panic buying or manufacturing strain during the pandemic, maybe. My MA has confessed she is totally out, others in the clinic then echoed, or confessed they had the same problem were nearly or almost out—and it's a struggle, Christmas, they have children... So, I use my lunch break to dash to Harmon's, a grocery store rumored online or on social media or some text thread—this is information from the MAs—to have toilet paper in stock. I buy four large packs—the limit, per customer—and as I walk out, fumble in my pockets, wishing I had cash for the bell ringer. The Salvation Army kettles. It seems unwise to me that they are doing the bell ringing, such a risk for infection, and does anyone really carry cash? I look up and see Charlene. She is the bell ringer. I can't believe it. This woman with metastatic cancer, who lives in the shelter, has bad lungs, bad hip—she is working as a bell-ringer?

I don't want to break any privacy rules, and I have to dash back to work anyway, afternoon clinic. But as soon as I can, I ask her about this—one might say I "chew her out."

"Charlene!" I say. "You of all people should not be doing that. You must have had to take a bus, another bus ride to get there, with all the infectious risks of that, and then all the people that come over to put something in the kettle, plus, just the standing with your hip, the time outside with your lungs and—"

She cuts me off. "Doc," she says. "You got to go to school, med school, train, whatever else so that then you can help me, all of us. I only went through ninth grade, I don't have money, I got to find the things I can do. I know the bus schedules by heart, I can ring a bell, I can smile. Even if I'm masked, people can see my eyes, and I can thank them. It's not much, what I do, the money in the kettle probably wouldn't buy one I-pill. But my life—everyone needs some way to help, to give back. You know?"

I did know. And marveled at her gratitude, positivity, goodness.

And, inevitably, Charlene's cancer stopped responding to treatment. Her oncologist didn't notify me, but they started hospice, and she moved to The Inn Between, a wonderful inpatient homeless hospice that looks like an apartment complex from the outside. It is actually not far from my home. I didn't know this until I saw her obituary.

I heard on the news that Dolly Parton, who had a song familiar to me, "Jolene," adapted it and called it "Vaccine." She sang it before she was vaccinated, and she donated a million dollars for the Covid-19 vaccine research. I love this, admire her greatly, am grateful. But I think Charlene instead, sing under my breath:

Charlene, Charlene, Charlene, Charlene
Your smile is like a breath of spring
Your voice is soft like summer rain
And I cannot compete with you, Charlene

Musical Interlude

When the pandemic started, I was studying with a piano professor at Westminster University, in Salt Lake City. She wanted nothing to do with online teaching, and I struggled to find someone open to this method of instruction. I cannot remember a time when I have not wanted to play the piano. For some reason the age at which I was supposed to start lessons was eight. I am not sure why. It may have been cost, but it seems, or seemed to my child mind, that there were many rules about what was allowed at what age, rules that lacked any sound reason. For example, age eight was also the proper age to have my ears pierced. And to be baptized. Though I think my ear piercings have closed over—I rarely wear jewelry—I did go for the piercing, I did wear a white dress and held my nose as I was tipped back and submerged in the baptismal font—at the age of eight. But with the piano—I really wanted to play. My sister is 16 months older than me, and when she started lessons, my asking became begging, cajoling, needling… and I started at age seven. My sister and I shared a teacher for a while, and I flew through music books, the multi-colored levels, each color determining higher levels of difficulty. Soon, after a year or two perhaps, my first teacher told my mother I had learned all she could teach me, and she, the teacher, took me to audition to become a student of Carol Hurst. Carol had been a piano instructor at Weber State University, and was the student of Fredrick Dickson, who was the student of Rafael Joseffi, who was the student of Franz Liszt.

She also was a former Miss Utah, and she and her husband were well-respected members of the community, part of the arts and educational establishment, philanthropic and talented. She was beautiful. Much later, I would see her without makeup, bald, in a bathrobe, having forgotten I was coming, in the midst of cancer treatment. And she was still stunningly beautiful. That first day I met her, however, and almost every other time, she had perfectly styled light blond hair, eye makeup, lipstick, she smelled wonderful, her posture straight, her gaze kind and scrutinizing. I do not remember what I played, and it cannot have been particularly good, but she took me on. As a student and—and as a person about whom she cared.

I loved Carol. I paid for my lessons, she charged a paltry sum, as she pointed out to me, $15 for 45 minutes, which usually stretched to an hour. It was not paltry to me. I had been working part time at my neighbor's needlepoint store since 6th grade, in addition to paper routes, baby-sitting, the usual girlhood jobs. This helped me pay for gymnastics and unexpected school expenses. But Carol's time was invaluable. To be in her home, sit near her, watch her, smell her, learn from her. I put a lot of time on schoolwork, was valedictorian in high school, and was determined to get a perfect ACT score and have a perfect 4.0 GPA. But I got up at 4AM to practice—my family piano was in a separate part of the house, and I kept the "soft pedal" down the whole time—but I am sure they suffered. Carol arranged for me to do a recital at the local arts center, with two other students. She played duos with me. She took me to concerts. She told me I was too thin, and my shoulders too hunched. She sang lyrics to the slow part when I played Chopin's Fantasie-Impromptu in C# minor. It was her favorite key, her red Cadillac license plate read CSHARP.

When I graduated from high school, Carol was no longer on faculty at the University. She suggested I take lessons from a former student of hers, so that I could use my scholarship money and, perhaps, do a music minor, knowing I planned to study medicine and most of my time would be needed for sciences. I did so for a semester or two.

Professor Nadine Bateman was excellent. Her method of teaching was very different from Carol's. I was required to memorize and play perfectly each measure of a piece, hands separately then together, before moving on to the next measure. I learned approximately 18 measures of Liszt's "Annee de Pelangre" in the entire year and played them flawlessly. Then, Nadine, as I was actually allowed to call her, died. She had lung cancer, having never smoked, stage IV at diagnosis, and fatal within months.

I also was increasingly required to focus on medicine, preparing for and taking the MCAT, then teaching MCAT prep courses, to help pay for medical school application, to pay rent to my mother. I switched to a chemistry minor. And still I played the piano, I always wanted to play. I often didn't—not feeling I could allow myself the luxury, having too much else to study, to do, clean, work. Carol recommended me for a Crystal Crest award at Weber State, she gave me a beautiful tapestry bag, covered in pianos. When I graduated she took me to local musicals.

In medical school, for a while, I didn't take lessons. Then I did. Carol allowed me to just telephone her—she never used email or computers, for that matter—and we would set up a time, she would suggest pieces. Then she too developed lung cancer. Like Nadine. Having never smoked. Her primary care doctor thinking she had allergies, then a cold, then maybe pneumonia then, finally, cancer. As a medical student, I learned all I could. She saw the lung specialist at my med school. She did chemotherapy, radiation, surgery. Was this somehow my fault? Was I toxic, two piano teachers, non-smokers, lung cancer?

One day, perhaps the day she had been in the bathtub when I came—I no longer came for lessons. I brought food. I watched *Jeopardy* with her and her husband, the still gorgeous Dean Hurst. She left me a voicemail that I still have. I hope. She says, "Melissa, this is Carol. Listen, I love you, you know that, I have always loved you. But I don't want to do lessons anymore. I can't. I want to just be friends. I hope that you understand. I will always love you…"

For about a decade after her death, I could not play Chopin's "Fantasie Impromptu," not for lack of practice, but because I would hear her singing, "I'm forever chasing rainbows…" with the rising, crescendo notes, then the descent. I don't know if she didn't know the words or was just needing to help me try to feel the emotion, but the words became da da da DAs, and I can feel the pressure of her hand on my forearm, leaning into the notes, the melody. It was too sad. I was too sad. I missed her too much. Another piece that forever I hear, in her alto voice, is "Autumn Leaves." "The autumn leeeeaaaaaves. Outside my winnnnndow..."

I bought my piano, the one I have now, about a year pre-pandemic. I had moved to my current home, on a sycamore-lined street East of Salt Lake City, relocating for my work at the inner-city clinic. It is a beautiful home, I worried about the cost, but Dr. Hardy rightly pointed out that it is an investment— "think of it as living in your bank." The old leaded-glass windows in the front room open out entirely, both panes push out like a fairytale house. The east windows in that room are stained glass, both from 1927, when it was built. The curved walls with cherry gumwood trim and the light wood floors seemed made for a piano—to hold it, the instrument and its sound—to reverberate and shape and warm the notes coming from the open lid.

When my piano arrived, the men bringing it placed it exactly where I asked. I had planned carefully, knowing I would be unlikely to move it easily. Later that evening, Kerwin from Dayne's Music came. Kerwin—I think of him as "Kerwin Daynes" though he is not—he is just the most wonderful piano salesperson in the world. He knew Carol and told me of a time when they had a shop in Ogden, and

Skip Daynes, the owner, felt they needed to close it, they were not making it. He called Carol Hurst to let her know, and she said "Now, Skippy…" And that same day she showed up at the store, and they sold two pianos that day. She sold them, I guess.

Kerwin brought with him some little covers for the piano's feet, and an "artist's bench" to replace the hard shiny black bench that came with the piano. He told me he thought Carol would want me to have it. The leather cushion was soft, the wheel to adjust the height moved easily. I tried to not cry. He showed me the best way to polish, to open and close the lid, told me that "Mr. Daynes" lived not far away, and he, Kerwin, stopped by of an evening not infrequently, so not to hesitate if I ever needed anything. For a moment, after he left, I sat on the bench, and I did cry. I felt I could smell the Upper Canada soap that forever reminded me of Carol. I avoid fragrance in general, overly sensitive, nausea… but this was cool and clean, sometimes with a hint of spearmint, her chewing gum, and I could hear, "chasing them da da deeeeeee. I'm forever chasing rainbows why oh why da da da da DEEE da da dum."

Eventually, I started lessons with Yu-Jane Yang, head of the piano department at Weber. I had asked her for a teacher recommendation, and she kindly took me on. She knew and loved Carol as well, we shared stories. Yu-Jane taught me in person, then when she spent summers in Taiwan with her aging and ailing mother, she taught me using Skype. This was perfect during later-pandemic. I tried to help with her mother, at least to answer questions, explain what the doctors might have meant. With Yu-Jane, I went to a music festival in Bavaria one summer. It was incredibly hot. The festival was for 2 weeks, and with my work, then as a hospitalist, I was only able to stay for one week. I had purchased one of the few remaining window fans in the village, and there was a bidding war for who would get it when I left. I played Mozart. At a piano festival. In Germany. This really happened. I have photos. Afterwards, we went to a gelato shop and sat outside, they had a 10-scoop dish, we each chose a flavor. I don't know if I ate any, but it was lovely. There is a photo. This did happen. I write that because it seems impossible, in the middle of clinic work, in the isolation and terror of a pandemic, in the knowledge that I haven't touched the piano in weeks... I tell myself it is true, look there, there is proof. The world is not only virus and you did play Mozart in Bavaria and go out for ice cream with other people.

I also visited the small industrial town where my great-grandfather was born, Zwickau, and Regensburg, the city where my grandfather was stationed during the war. I had a minor accident in my rental car. I got sick. But those things are not part of a musical interlude. They just made those magical moments even more so.

Yu-Jane understandably expects a significant dedication from her students, and with my move to Salt Lake and difficult work in clinic, I found myself not able to devote enough time. My Westminster teacher was more casual, but then… pandemic. I have no teacher currently but have possibilities. I have tried some lessons with a wonderful Eastern European musician. We have met on Zoom or, pandemic permitting, masked and in person. I hope that I do not, somehow, give her lung cancer. I told her that I want to learn all the Beethoven Sonatas, and that is all I want to play, and although she initially recommended—as perhaps a good teacher must—exploring a broader more well-rounded repertoire, she acceded to my plan.

She assigned me reading, Beethoven's letter to his brothers, the Heiligenstadt Testament. I am not sure why but reading it I felt a certain affinity with this man. Not that I have any musical talent, or anything like his degree of genius in any field. Such pain and tragedy to be losing his hearing, needing, or feeling a need to hide it, even as he is beginning to be known as a skilled composer. Being perceived as angry, withdrawn, when in fact needing to conceal his deafness led to his solitude. And certainly fear, pain, depression must have weighed him down and led to isolation. I wonder if there is something in that isolation that made his music most compelling, at a time when the world was in lock-down, when isolation became a necessity in order to avoid COVID, to be able to continue my work, see patients, avoid spreading a deadly virus.

But also, knowing that I am not well. And having to conceal that, must all doctors do that? In order to care for patients and be at all credible, must I not project health, or at the very least be neutral in this regard, not have my own health or illness anywhere in the room or the clinic, but cloaked in my white coat, to hear and to heal, if possible, then disappearing home, to learn whatever I can, to read, study, think, and grapple with my own health struggles, alone. And for Beethoven, did he have, perhaps, a black cloak, going out to play, conduct, hear-but-not hear his pieces performed, then retreat into solitude, to think, compose, hide?

But knowing only vague bits regarding his deafness, depression, I had wanted to play these Sonatas. Why? I am not sure, but perhaps his turmoil is there in the music, even without the facts. The beauty, the despair. The raging and the concealing. The rests between storms. In the *Fourth Sonata, Op.7 No.4*, I can play along, repeated notes in the left hand, ascending triplets for the right, *Allegro con Brio*, and yet underneath, there is something, beneath the brightness. There, then in the *Largo con gran Espressione* it surfaces, sadness, loss, each measure heartbreakingly slow, two notes, then equal length rests, then the next measure the same, two beautiful, poignant notes, and the equivalent pause.

But also, with the Beethoven sonatas, it is a plan, always so appealing. No thought required regarding what piece to play. I play Beethoven sonatas. My teacher helps me decide which to learn, what technique exercises will be best, which order, what tempo for practice, and, since I get dreadfully nervous at lessons, she typically plays along with me. Though in my heart I know it quite unlikely I will manage to learn them all, impossible, I can for now pretend, just play.

Rockstar, my Aussie of endless energy, sleeps under the piano when I play. Maybe he feels I am safe, knows where I am and can rest from his work of shepherding me, letting Beethoven take a turn at quelling the demons. I don't practice nearly enough. But I always want to. Working, charting, studying, cleaning, sorting, exercising, all else, it seems, must be done first, and then the day is running out and so—so music gets pushed back, afternoon, evening, next day. I am a doctor, a physician, not a musician, so this is okay. The piano sits grandly, waiting. The bench height is mine, and on it lies the Teflon silver Sundance vest given to me by Dr. Hardy, when one day I came to an appointment foolishly underdressed for the cold. When I cannot manage, when Air Fairy is raging, when it does not feel possible to hold together, I put it on, zip it up, sit on the artist's bench from Kerwin, set a metronome, stroke the white stripe that stretches from the tip of Rockstar's nose to between his ears at the top of his head, and then begin with scales.

Diagnosis: Triangle

Gretchen tells me that she is concerned about a blood vessel on her stomach. There has been a blizzard, and I am working from my home office—well, from my home. In truth, I move around, move my laptop to various spots. Sometimes a different window, a new view, I think, will help me see things more clearly, broaden my differential diagnosis—or maybe I am just stir-crazy. I am currently working from my living room, standing at my old wooden drop-down desk, looking out the leaded glass front windows at the storybook neighborhood covered in snow. My laptop and a cup of blueberry tea on a coaster rest on the closed desktop. Gretchen is in her apartment, meeting with me via video. As the months of pandemic continued, our clinic, medicine, doctors, me—we've improved and increased our use of technology to enable virtual visits—platforms that protect patient privacy. Technology to allow me to send a patient a text message, then call her if I don't "see" her joining me, tell her to allow access to her cell phone's video and camera. This has been useful in this winter of record-breaking snow.

Gretchen says she feels there is an electrical sort of shock, like a wire of pain. She is concerned because she thinks it looks like a triangle. I don't understand what she means. She is unmasked, naturally, she is alone. She doesn't have teeth. I forget this when I see her in clinic, masked. It must be hard to eat. How easy it is to forget how easy my life is in so many ways. Absence of teeth does not seem to make it hard to smoke, and Gretchen puffs on, sometimes struggling to quit, sometimes struggling to want to quit. Too expensive. But too anxious.

Too bored.

"A triangle?" I ask.

She lies back on her bed and lifts her shirt, then by moving her cell phone around a bit, with my navigation help—"a little more to the left…" she shows me her abdomen, left mid-low region. I cannot see anything that looks like a triangle, or in any way pathologic, and I tell her I think things look okay. She feels there is something there. We decide to get an ultrasound.

The radiology scheduling office calls, and my staff send me a message.

"What are you looking for with the ultrasound? Need more details. Abdomen and Pelvis? Transvaginal? Doppler/Aorta?"

I do not think I can write "rule out triangle," and my initial reason, "left-sided abdominal pain" is apparently inadequate. They somehow decide to "rule out hernia."

I see Gretchen in clinic a week or so later, a less blizzard-y day. We review the ultrasound report.

"The radiologist says no evidence of hernia," I say.

"I didn't think I had a hernia," she says.

"Neither did I," I say. "But it also seems nothing else problematic was noted—it looked pretty much normal." She is not reassured.

"I feel there is something in there, something was implanted." She looks a little hesitant.

"Implanted when, by whom?" I ask.

"People think I am crazy," she is a bit tearful. "But I was abducted by aliens, and I saw my brain, and it was golden. I know I am one of the 47,000 chosen, noted in the *Book of Revelations*, to help the earth transition. I have Heavenly Father's blood in me."

I am really cautious in my reply. Gretchen has mentioned conspiracy theories, some related to COVID vaccines—which she has consistently refused to take. She feels she is being poisoned at her apartment or damaged by microwaves. But this seems a bit more vivid or—something. I am not a psychiatrist and don't really know what it is.

I do know that her diabetes is not controlled. She refuses to take any medicines, pills. She will use one type of insulin, though she periodically stops taking even this, usually for unclear reasons. At least unclear to me. She then becomes more sick, exhausted, has more neuropathic pain, loses weight. And thinks that is due to the toxic apartment complex, or to radio waves, or to her boyfriend having gotten vaccinated and then having sex with her. Etc. Recently, she needed to renew her driver's license, and her blood sugar has been out of control, dangerously so. Without her checking it, I fear it is high or low, particularly as she eats sporadically, and gives herself insulin based upon how she feels, not on any glucose lab data. I tell her I am not comfortable signing her form. If I sign it, that would be indicating that her diabetes is under control. It isn't, and I don't feel it is safe for her to drive. We agree that if she can faithfully check and record her glucoses daily, show that they are indeed stable, that she can achieve a level of management that will make it safe for her to drive without harm to herself or someone else, I will fill out her form. She commits to doing this for two weeks.

Unfortunately, she didn't do it. She lost her notebook, she left it home, her cat distracted her. All probably true. Also, she doesn't like to think about being diabetic and doesn't like having to face it, doesn't believe sometimes that it is a problem, or a reality.

After relating what she meant, the implantation, abduction, and so on, she asks if I think she is crazy, if I believe her.

I say, “Well, there are a lot of things I don’t understand.”

She suggests I read the *Bible*, the *Book of Revelations*.

I ask her if God would want her to lie, and if not, why she didn’t do her glucose log and insulin as she had agreed. I am not sure if this is terrible, psychologically or morally, so I ask Dr. Hardy about it, later. He thinks it is sort of clever, I think, and that the patient, Gretchen, has a delusional disorder. I start to describe some of our encounter, not unkindly but perhaps with too much “Can you believe this?” in my voice. Then, kindly, he reminds me of my own craziness.

“Spiders in the arse. Air Fairy.” Code words. Right.

Back to Gretchen. After we discuss her glucose log, she tells me, again, that she will not take the COVID vaccine. I try to decide whether to discuss it today, always spoken to Dragon, documented in my notes as “vaccine refused, counseling provided,” as though that absolves me if she gets sick and I failed to be convincing enough. Or I failed to present the data well or—or something. But counseling has been provided many times, and I am not sure if there is more to be gained today. Perhaps just focusing on the blood sugars is most important. Then she tells me that she bought some diatomaceous earth online, and that if she gets COVID, she can take that, or she might even take small amounts now, to prevent it. I tell her I don’t think that is a good plan, I advise against it. But we can talk about COVID again and any other concerns she has next visit. Counseling provided.

In Sickness and in Health, Till Death Do Us Part

As I pulled off his right sock, I realized, to my horror, that a large portion of my patient's great toe had come off as well. It was inside the sock, I was certain, but I did not want to take it out.

"Oh," I said, brilliantly.

It was late afternoon, or well into the evening, really. I had been about to leave the clinic, when the PSRs—Patient Services Representatives—sent an electronic message asking if I could just quickly see a Navajo man just for medication refills. His name was Bahe. The astute reader will recognize his appearance in this book earlier. But here I want to show more of my initial interaction with him, and highlight his devotion to his wife, who we know as well, Anna. Bahe had not been seen at the clinic before, so he would need an appointment: I had to see him in order for him to get medications from our pharmacy. I suspect if I had just asked the PSR to send me a telephone message in the EMR, electronic medical record, with the medications needed and then had them get him scheduled with me in the next few weeks, no one would have argued. In any case, Bahe, it seemed, was unsure about what medicines he was on. The PSRs messaged me that they knew only that he was diabetic. And it turned out that not only had he not been seen in our clinic before, it seemed he had not had medical care elsewhere, anywhere, for several years—all of which made a visit truly necessary.

I confess to a rather hefty sigh, unheard except by Rockstar, who dutifully yawned and went back to sleep in his kennel in the corner of my office. It had been a full day, I was tired. But that is wrong. What else did I have to do that mattered? Tired is wrong. I have no children, no spouse, what else do I have to do? Devotion to work, dedication to medicine, or Air Fairy? In any case, I set down my backpack and re-donned my white coat. Still masked—typically I leave my N95 mask on until I am in my car after work and heading home—I waited for my MA, Lindy, to quickly check in and room the patient. I thanked her, apologized for keeping her late.

I knock on the door then go in. Bahe is not yet 40, I know from his chart, but he, and his wife who sits beside him, look closer to 60. Their skin is dark and lined, their once-dark hair is graying, their hands are callused, fingernails dirty. And they beam. Their eyes smile, gleam, above their pale blue surgical masks.

"Hi, I say. "I'm Dr. Bentley. Bahe?"

"Hi, doc," he says, "thanks so much for seeing me, I know it's kind of late. We just were nearby and saw the clinic and had heard about it, a clinic free for Natives, and I've been out of my diabetes meds for a while so we just stopped by."

"That's great." I reply. "Where have you been seen for your diabetes, do you have another doctor you usually see? What medicines are you on? How are your blood sugars?"

I kick myself mentally for asking four questions at once. It is overwhelming and does not save time.

"Well, I went to the clinic at Ft. Hall for an eye exam, I think they did blood, when was that?" he says turning to his wife.

"Well, it's been a few years now…" she speaks quietly and I suspect she knows the year, if not the exact date. Perhaps she is reluctant to admit to not having seen a doctor for a while, as though that is some sort of failing on her or their part?

“Okay. What is your name?” I say.

“Anna.”

“Okay. Are you taking any medicines right now, or using insulin?”

The answer to this is shaking heads, both of them answering for him, I assume. I suggest we do some lab work to check his diabetes control, a hemoglobin A1c which will give me an idea of his average blood sugar for the past approximately 3 months. I will get him a new glucometer and supplies to check his blood sugar each morning and a logbook to write it down, along with anything else—I ask him to keep track of especially active days, or if he has just eaten a box of Twinkies, or if he has forgotten to take his medication one day—anything that might explain glucose readings that seem aberrant. We plan on starting with metformin, a usual diabetes medication that should not cause low blood sugars, something that worries them both. We also plan to check cholesterol, kidney function, a few other things, and to have him back soon. I listen to his heart and lungs. There is so much more—when was that eye exam? Blood pressure, urine protein, vaccinations—but I tell myself I will see him soon. Again, don’t overwhelm: self or patient.

“Is there anything else, does that sound okay, make sense?” I ask. Three questions. Argh.

“What about her, my wife?” Bahe asks.

And it turns out that Anna is also diabetic, and so I have her added on to the schedule as well, so I can place orders, labs, medications, glucometer, document, I listen to her history, her heart and lungs.

Almost stopping myself, reluctant, tired, I ask again “Is there anything else, all set?” Two or even 1.5 questions; better.

Anna nudges her husband and says something almost inaudible, but

I catch the word "foot" and then she says more loudly, "You should show her your foot."

Bahe says nothing, so I say, "Can I see your feet?"

He unlaces his work boots, they seem sort of molded to his feet, his socks are stained the tan color of the shoes and a darker rusty color at the toes of that right foot. He has a hard time reaching his feet, had managed to unlace the shoes and use his other foot to get each off, but I help him by taking off the socks—and the toe.

There is a podiatrist in clinic, but only once a week and by now it is too late to ask him to come in. I use some of the podiatry supplies, iodoform, loose sterile gauze—but the toe, the foot, is clearly infected, and my own rule of thumb—or toe—is that if I can see the bone, it is osteomyelitis, bone infection. I worry that he will become septic, have overwhelming and possibly fatal bloodstream infection, and that he will lose his whole foot.

I attempt to find the right balance in conveying this to Bahe and Anna. It is very serious. But manageable, can be treated, I can help. I give him an antibiotic shot. By this time, I have some lab results, his glucose is over 500, he has an elevated white blood cell count, possibly suggesting infection, he has ketones, which suggests acidosis. With all of this, I tell him he needs to go to the hospital.

"We don't have insurance," he says.

"I know," I say. "It's okay."

I tell them how to get to the University ER, close by, they don't want transport, Anna will drive. I send Lindy home, then call the ER, speak to the triage/intake nurse, and fax my quickly dictated notes and the results I have so far. I am glad, mostly, to have looked at his foot. That "mostly"—how awful I have become! He might have lost his foot, even died. I look at Rockstar, who is fine. We head for home. I'm just that tired.

I am not and have not ever been married. So, I have no right to write about the institution of marriage. Even my own parents were divorced when I was seven. No insights from inside the partnership, the family. But what I do have, as so often it seems, are observations from inside my white coat, seeing patients, couples, husbands and wives. Occasional same-sex partnerships. Sometimes both partnered are my patients, sometimes just one. When I see a particular patient, Hugh, who is a retired judge/rancher, who has heart disease, diabetes, liver disease, bone marrow disease, osteoarthritis, asthma, insomnia, depression—his wife comes, or is present on the virtual video screen, always. We consider her our "consultant." A term Hugh first used, as she typically had information or a perspective she felt it was necessary to share with me, and he either valued her contribution or had resigned himself to hearing it anyway.

Another case in which I saw one member of a couple was Hatem. He was nearing 40 as well, had immigrated from Iraq where he was a policeman, perhaps 10 years earlier. He smoked, a lot, and had high cholesterol, borderline diabetes, and very high blood pressure. I saw him monthly, he required B12 shots each month for neuropathy and pernicious anemia. Every time I saw him, his blood pressure was high. Eventually, he was on five medications, all different classes, that should have worked synergistically. And I was doing laboratory assessments for rare causes of resistant hypertension; things like unusual tumors, vascular narrowing, genetic disorders. I went over his medications again and again, was he taking them? What time? We worked on low sodium diet. Nothing seemed to get his blood pressure down. I checked with the pharmacy, and he did pick up his medications each month. During the pandemic, I was able to get him a blood pressure cuff and had him keep monitoring at home, thinking maybe it was high due to nerves in the clinic, "white coat hypertension," though he did not seem anxious with me. And I did not think that could account for it being so very high.

Hatem did not like the virtual visits, and usually was not visible on video, but agreed to talking on the phone. With an interpreter, I checked in with him.

“Hi, Hatem. How are you?”

“Good,” he replied. He did speak a fair bit of English.

“Have you stopped smoking yet?”

He laughed.

“No, doctora—” then started in Arabic.

“He says he is too stressed right now, he can’t go anywhere, he got in a fight and now has legal issues and can’t go visit his family in Iraq unless the judge drops the case and so he has to go outside to smoke,” Ali, the interpreter relates.

“Hmm,” I say. “That sounds bad. You shouldn’t get in fights and you shouldn’t smoke.” Yes, years of med school and residency and study and that is my great wisdom.

“Are you taking the bupropion?” I ask. This is a medicine he has told me was helping, it is used both for smoking cessation and for depression/anxiety.

“Yes. 300mg each morning,” he says.

“Okay. How is your blood pressure?”

He gives me numbers which I double check with the interpreter—they are so high. 190/100, 200/95, 185/95… This is even worse than before, when in clinic.

“Those are high.” All that training. “Are you taking your medications?”

I am sure I have asked that before, but maybe I have just gone over them, made sure he had them and knew what they were, when to take them. Because if he wanted to lie to me, he could have made up good blood pressure readings. Or maybe he just feels able to tell me something on the phone that he couldn't in person.

Hatem says something in Arabic. Ali interprets: "He gives most of his medicine to his wife, because they have been checking her blood pressure and it is really high."

"You can't do that," I say, partly telling it to myself as well, as I feel such concern for Hatem, his wife, this little family. "It is against the law, and you need the medicines, they are ordered for you, your blood pressure is too high. With smoking, cholesterol, borderline diabetes, I worry about you having a heart attack or a stroke," I say.

Ali interprets, Hatem replies in Arabic. Interpretation: "I'm sorry, doctor, but my responsibility is to take care of my wife. She is the most important and I will continue to give it to her."

I ask about whether she could make an appointment, or doesn't she have a doctor, could she see her doctor? Hatem seems to be done talking for now, and schedules another appointment, in a month, though he isn't coming in person and I would like to check on his blood pressure sooner.

He misses the appointment. I worry. It is unlike him to "no-show" or not answer the phone for his appointments. I am able to access the electronic health records for the University hospital from my clinic. As the primary care physician, I am able to do so legally, even if I am not caring for the patient while he is in hospital. I check to see if Hatem has been seen. He has. It's hard to tell, scrolling through notes, visits, imaging reports, but I think he is still there. And has been for weeks. Could that be true? It could, it is. He had a stroke.

There are two broad categories of stroke, ischemic, in which an area of the brain tissue doesn't get blood for a time, due to a thrombus, moving clot, or a blocked vessel, for example. This is by far the most common, and can be very damaging, especially in certain areas of the brain. It also can sometimes be very successfully treated by directly removing the clot or opening the vessel with a surgical procedure or with thrombolytics—clot busting medications. The other more rare and devastating type of stroke is hemorrhagic. The problem then is not lack of blood, but too much, a bleed into the brain. Brain bleeds often occur with trauma, but a hemorrhagic stroke is the dreaded outcome of uncontrolled severe high blood pressure, which can burst vessels in the brain. And this is what happened to Hatem.

I think, reading through the chart, neuro ICU notes, and records, that he will die. He doesn't. He goes to inpatient rehab. He goes home. Eventually, vaccinated and masked, he comes to see me, his son pushing him in a wheelchair.

"Hi," I say. He smiles, lopsided.

"Have you stopped smoking?" I ask.

He laughs. I want to cry. The left upper ¼ of his cranium is caved in, it looks squishy. Eventually he'll have additional neurosurgery. They evacuated the bleed from that area, and they try to create a somewhat more rounded skull, later. I wonder if I should have prescribed even more blood pressure medications. So he could share. I had wondered if I should document that he was giving them to his wife, I couldn't remember if I did, and if, then—well, the clinic has a pharmacy and our patients get medications at no cost to them, but it is subsidized by the IHS and CMS—Medicaid and Medicare—and I cannot prescribe medications for people I am not seeing—then we would lose our licensing and then no patients could get them. I won the Ethics Prize, remember... so what I did must have been right. If only.

I later meet Hatem's wife, virtually. She has many questions and requests, letters, so that she can be paid for caring for him, supplies such as adult diapers, shower chairs, to be delivered, "all medications refilled" without knowing what those medicines are—including those from the neurologist whom he was supposed to see for follow-up. Supposed to, but didn't, didn't have a ride, didn't know the location—something. She looks kind, devoted, is beautiful. Beloved by her husband, devastatingly so.

Another instance when I was the doctor for a husband, I did not meet his wife, but it showed something else about marriage. Or love, I suppose. I find, again from inside a white coat, not from inside the union, that there are as many versions of it—marriage, love—as there are people. Variations, ways of caring or not, ways of living as partners or not. Ways in which the marriage, the two people united help each other achieve greater health, or not. But also I find that qualities of a person seen by a spouse may not be otherwise obvious. The front put on for society, or for a doctor, may hide a great deal of what a person really is, means, feels.

Gary saw me only once before the pandemic. He was in his 60s, gray hair and gray skin and gray clothes. He also smoked, did not want to work on quitting, he only smoked outside, so it didn't hurt anyone else. He had chronic back pain, for which he wanted me to prescribe oxycontin. He had not recently seen a doctor, but when he last did, this was what was prescribed.

I told him I was sorry that he was in pain, and that I did not think this was a necessarily safe or good medicine or good way to treat chronic pain. I suggested a more thorough evaluation, possible orthopedic consult, figuring out the cause, working with physical therapy, turmeric, lidocaine patch, topical voltaren gel.

He was underwhelmed or mistrustful of my sorrow for his pain and seemed dismissive of my suggestions. In any case, his expression was hostile or, at best, shut-down, his voice angry or dissatisfied, or tired or—some combination. As I went through my usual internal medicine new patient visit—he did not want to do colon cancer screening or have his cholesterol checked or be screened for diabetes. He was willing to start taking a blood pressure medicine he had been on before, and to schedule follow-up. He seemed annoyed.

I did not think he would keep his follow-up appointment, and he did miss one or two, but then he scheduled and came, masked, to get vaccinated for COVID. He agreed to refill his blood pressure medicine. He told me then—I should have known before, did I not ask, take a thorough social history? He told me that his wife had advanced multiple sclerosis, MS, and that he worried if she got COVID she would die. Gary took care of her, fed her, bathed her, was not willing to let anyone else come in, home health aides, for fear they would bring the virus. I would like to have been able to say that would not happen, but I know that it did, it does. Instead, I tell him I am very glad he is getting vaccinated and I hope he will take care of himself for her sake, since she needs him. Maybe stop smoking?

The next time I see him I actually hear him first, as I knock, then open the exam room door: he roars. He is so. Very. Angry.

"Goddamn fucking bastards, they let her die, she died like a dog, a dog would have had a better life and death. You did it, you took her, you goddamn fucking doctors, took her away and she died like a dog..."

I did not say anything. I sat. I listened. Eventually he told me what happened.

His wife had choked, aspirated, wasn't breathing. He called 911, she was taken to the hospital, they told him she had pneumonia and needed help breathing, and then she wasn't strong enough to go home, but they needed the hospital bed, he said. So, they sent her to a nursing home. With COVID precautions, he was not allowed to visit, she could not talk on the phone, he could not see her.

He called every day to see how she was and was told she was fine. Until one day he was told she had COVID. It was spreading through the facility.

He called every day, he was told she was stable. Until one day he was told to come, and he did, and she had died.

Inexplicably—but what made any sense, what was explainable in this time?—he was allowed to go into her room. And it seemed nothing had been done, meaning that he found her naked, covered in urine, feces, sweat, sprawled on a bare mattress.

When he had choked out this story, heartbreakingly, Gary cried. He sobbed. He had taken off his mask, had been shouting, spluttering, and now this soft crying, nose streaming. I should have moved close, taken his hand. And yet. And yet—COVID—and I did not want to spread it, to be unable to work. I handed him another box of tissues. I listened to him sob for a long time. I held him with my eyes. Then we were quiet.

Shepherd Spring

Bounding the deck, his white paws marvelous-mudded-lick-kissable as salted chocolate, the dark earth gorgeous after months of grueling white and gray—my Aussie hurls his hoary harvest towards me, scarcely pausing to breathe, pant, another lap, making a path, circling, round and round and round the dappled yard.

It is not spring, just an early melt. Barely have we crept, cautiously, peered palely out of our home-burrows to find whether that bit of robin noise is a hallucinating ear, a dream, or real life starting again cracking gorgeous blue sky, with a sun finally bright enough for shadows, but also maybe warmth.

And here is revealed what my dog has been planting all along the cold months; whilst I scoured seed books he labored on, never ceased, digging through layers of ice and snow. His harvest then: a glorious hot pink elephant, raised from an icy grave, flung skyward, then squeaking in desperation as its middle is chomped; eight or twelve mittens, possibly four are mine, none have their mates. I say a silent prayer of apology, Forgive me sad stranger, you with one cold hand, doomed to go about unmatching. Elsewhere, a similar sock-sown patch. And in one wonderful corner carved into the ice-earth, bones of all sorts, in quantity to construct a sizable herd, though only their legs. I feel a bit gruesome, ghost cow legs wandering the frozen walks, but the butcher had assured me they ate grass and were doomed to die whether I bought the bones or no.

My dog pauses, sheer amazement at the goodness, CAN YOU BE-

LIEVE THIS, bursting, his laugh-pant, such joy, gorgeous brown eyes gazing up, hind quarters shaking with delight.

I know, my pretty friend, I say. It's unimaginable, you've no words to bear it. And neither have I.

Singing bowls

I felt, more than heard, the tone, from the bowl, low and soft, from somewhere near the front of the room, I could not see. At first it was—well, I felt calmer, which is impressive, given that I was very worried about the not-gone pandemic, the crowd of people sitting around me, the paucity of masks. Unused as I was to gathering in-person with anyone, any number of people together would seem a lot, I suppose, but this truly was such. Row after row of chairs in the large hotel ballroom, all occupied, people, mouths, breath, words, handshakes and hugs even. Could it be safe? And then, as the chatter around me continued, I felt anxious about that—the chatter, the noise, the lack of awareness—we were now integrative medicine practitioners—should we not be coming to attention, tuning in, listening, resonating?

Mimi Guarneri used the soft hammer against the lip of the blue crystal bowl, once again, then ran it around the crystal rim. It took a moment, but the sound, hum, tone seemed to thrum inside my chest, vibrate alongside my heart. I sat at the back of the large auditorium. Dr. Guarneri is a cardiologist, and had spent much of her career putting stents into hearts, before deciding to try to help those hearts earlier, before the vessels, valves, electrical pathways were damaged. She also decided that 80-100-hour work weeks, scant and scattered chances to eat, sleep, see friends or family was not, actually, healthy. Was not sustainable, for her. But then, looking more broadly, the system of "care" in which she was participating was not sustainable for other people either—her colleagues, the country, the planet. Now, she is the President of the Academy of Integrative Health and Medicine, AIHM, and was playing the singing bowl in front of the annual conference. My class, "Cohort 9," was graduating. Our Integrative Medicine Fellowship graduation ceremony—the culmination of two years of coursework, study, testing, training—was to take place as part of this conference.

Instead of growing silent however, readying for the speaker, people enthusiastically exchanged greetings, even, yes, hugs—surely not safe. It was a bit remarkable to see my cohort, the 18 people with whom I had spent hours on Zoom, and no time in person, until now. They were short! And tall! And real! Somehow Zoom windows, at times, became cartoonish, these squares with faces inside talking or listening or eating or forgetting to mute and yelling at a child who was yelling at a sibling, or forgetting to unmute, something I sometimes just took for granted, reading lips unthinkingly, until someone else remembered the microphone icon, unmute. But they were actually whole bodies, whole people. And undoubtedly others at the conference knew and had not seen each other for a while: there was a lot to talk about. But still. Be still.

I had started the fellowship in October of 2020, the first year of the pandemic. "The interested reader"—I think of my Dragon macro/command, for dictating HPI—the history of the present illness—in charts for patients with endless complicated medical conditions, stories— "The interested reader is referred to prior notes for complete history…" is what my note would read. Was there ever such an interested reader? Were any of my notes actually read, not simply scanned for complexity/medical decision-making to meet billing codes?

But in this case, I was about to write only that an interested reader could refer to my fellowship scholarship application for details about my reason for pursuing this training. Here, I will simply write that traditional Western Medicine seemed to be failing on several fronts. I didn't know what to do to help my patients during the pandemic. With COVID, before vaccines and treatments, other than addressing their pre-existing/chronic medical conditions, which may make them more susceptible to illness and to more severe illness, what could I, their trusted doctor, offer? And it seemed that lifestyle or just life circumstances, style be damned, were key: poverty, low quality food, polluted air, mental illness, lack of exercise, substance use/addiction, lack of access to regular preventive/primary health care. On and on. What should I prescribe for these ailments? I think some patients shared my disillusionment with pharmaceuticals—advertising, side effects, huge profits for drug companies, interactions, polypharmacy. And the very process of delivering "health care" within the system was contributing to the degradation of the planet, soil, air, water—that then made patients sicker, that then led to more health care use... And that seemed an endless cycle. My patients: American Indian/Alaskan Native, people experiencing homelessness, refugees, as well as the very old, with complicated compound medical conditions—were the most vulnerable. To climate change, to COVID, to life struggles, to death.

In any case, this seemed an opportunity to look for a less harmful way to practice. To, "first do no harm." I wanted to try to learn the wisdom of other healing traditions, and to focus on true health, dis-ease, think both more broadly and more deeply about illness, about the art and science of medicine.

I did not first encounter singing bowls in the context of Healing Sound within Integrative Medicine. It was at a concert at the Cathedral of the Madeline, an astonishing Gothic Cathedral near Capitol Hill in Salt Lake City. Unlike the iconic Mormon Temple, gleaming white and prominent downtown and in tourist advertising, the Cathedral of the Madeline is tucked away, its grandeur subtle, but then startling. Walking the street, one might notice the front staircase, then eyes moving upwards, see the ornately carved wooden doors. Then the lancet windows, then the rose windows atop, and then, view spreading up and out, the astonishing carvings, stone ornamentation, more windows until, finally, eyes reach the edges of the massive structure: the spires pointing skyward. The massive structure—trying to take it all in, leaning back further and further, one is thrown off balance.

Inside, the cathedral is differently astonishing: there is nothing subtle, it is just glorious. Walls muraled with biblical figures, painted in wild colors along every space of plaster, and, interspersed, stained glass. Gleaming gold trim, candles, sculpture, light.

The concert at which I saw and heard singing bowls was performed by the Utah Chamber Artists, a remarkable choir that, uniquely I think, intersperses sopranos, altos, tenors, basses—rather than grouping them by section. Their voices blend, and stand out, at the same time, the individual qualities and the perfect harmony. In this concert, the percussion section used crystal bowls from Hawaii, using a mallet to strike the side and to slide around the rims, creating that reverberation, resonance. The bowls glowed in the stage light, the faces of the musicians too seemed to shine, until at the end, all lights were extinguished, the sound slowly fading. Then the full cathedral was pregnant with perfect silence, that lasted. Almost eerily, probably less than a minute, and yet longer, infinitely. Before an eruption of applause and approbation, bows, encores, and cheer.

Now though, at the fellowship graduation conference, it is the healing properties of the crystal bowls, rather than their astounding beauty, that is of paramount importance, as I relate to Dr. G., her preferred form of address.

"Crystal Harmonics, 100%," she is saying.

I have asked her, consulted her, for Dr. Hardy. I have tried to convey how Dr. Hardy has, is, perpetually, saving my life, through the pandemic, and for years before. How he makes it possible for me to work, to be a doctor, to try to help my patients, the only thing I can do that maybe matters, and to try—to try to be a person, to have hope to—to manage, fight Air Fairy, allow myself to sit and to eat and sleep and want things, and...

And I try to convey this without actually saying, "Air Fairy" or seeming so entirely crazy that Dr. G. immediately rescinds my fellowship credentials and commits me to the psych hospital.

"It is his heart," I have said. I give Dr. Guarneri some details about the pathology, the problem, trying to be concise. And also, I don't know all the details because Dr. Hardy has not told me.

What I don't tell Dr. G is that I keep remembering a horrific experience from residency. It was my first rotation, as an intern, having completed four years of medical school, almost all in a classroom, and knowing nothing practical, it seemed. I was assigned to the cardiac critical care unit, the CCU, at the largest hospital in the city. A patient had undergone a MAZE procedure, a process of isolating problematic electrical activity in the heat that can trigger atrial fibrillation or atrial flutter. Then the problematic patch of heart is burned, cauterized, killed—then the normal pathway of electrical activity, orderly, from the normal physiologic "pacemaker," the SA node, across the atrial to the AV node, then into the ventricles through the bundle of His, bundle branches, and Purkinje fibers. This at least I know, from texts, from tests. However, my first overnight call, this patient post-procedure bled—there had been inadvertent burning through the heart to the aorta, the main blood vessel that carries blood to the entire body. The patient bled to death, as I tried desperately to get help, the fellow, the attending cardiologist, anyone in the hospital who knew what to do. And also, as I tried to stay awake, horrified at myself for being sleepy as someone was dying

And now—though again, I am not sure of the details—I imagine that Dr. Hardy's heart condition is similar. He is to undergo surgery, he has let me know, and I will not see him for a week. It is not his first heart surgery or procedure. And now I do know a bit more than I did as an intern—but still do not know what to do. I am not his doctor, fortunately, because I am not a cardiologist or cardiothoracic surgeon. But unfortunately too, because I cannot imagine any doctor caring about him as much as I do. I would do anything to help him. And so I think of the healing crystal bowls.

"The F, heart chakra," Dr. G. is saying.

I find a bowl, in a lovely blue, my favorite color—I do not know what Dr. Hardy's favorite color is, so cannot look for that. The bowl I choose has abalone shell, ecologically sound, found shells, like those I collected when escaping, mid-pandemic, to the place Dr. Hardy found, near Mendocino. A place of respite and magic, where there was a farm and humming llamas and headlands—and abalone shells. I order the bowl for Dr. Hardy from Crystal Harmonics, and it arrives, and I give it to him, as a Christmas gift, but really as a healing gift. It is something to do, I hope, I pray, to help, prior to his surgery, and in the weeks after. Maybe, somehow, the tone will resonate, heal the rhythm, the discordance, whatever is awry in his heart tissues. Maybe, somehow, I can atone for my prior failure as a tired inexperienced intern. I am so afraid Dr. Hardy will die, my punishment for not only not knowing what to do that long ago day in the CCU, but for also, even, horribly, struggling just to stay awake. And countless lifelong failings, sins of omission and commission, weakness, selfishness. Not knowing, not paying attention, taking too much—time, space, everything.

I wrap the singing bowl for Dr. Hardy, so carefully, and deliver it. I intend to include a little message that was on the invoice, something in Hawaiian, I think, though I confess I don't know. I hope it is a healing message, which is a bit silly, I suppose. But I want, of course, to cut off the price. It was expensive, but I would have spent any amount I could, if it would help at all.

And Dr. Hardy is so kind, even without me telling him about it, at first, the meaning of the bowl, the connection to the past, the fear I have. He knows, I think, how or why I have given him this gift. He says he cannot accept it. I plead, explain then, about having consulted Dr. G., his heart, the healing, the fellowship, the abalone, the heart chakra, the concert at the Cathedral of the Madeline, which Dr. Hardy also attended, with the bowls there. Christmas. My fear he will die. My helplessness. Please, please, please keep it, I plead.

I have to return to the Mayo clinic for six-month follow-up, having undergone brain surgery in March. Since it is December, I suppose it is a bit more than six months, but a nice time, weatherwise, to be in Phoenix. While I am there, Dr. Hardy and I communicate via email, and when I return, his surgery is done, and he arranges a time for me to pick up the bowl. It is snowy for a while, and hard to get anywhere, so there is a bit of delay, during which I hope that he will reconsider, Please, please, please. I ask if I can give it as a gift to his wife, who of course is worried about him too. But I recognize that I need to respect his decision, finally, and do pick it up. I feel, again, that I have failed, I still do not know what to do. It sits in a box in my basement. I cry. A lot. But Dr. Hardy didn't die during surgery.

For a while, I think maybe if I don't sleep, now, somehow that can atone for the past. But I can't manage that for long, and fear it will impact my clinic work, and know, logically, it is not of any use. I tell Dr. Hardy about the patient who died in the CCU when I was an intern. I tell him what he already knows, and has helped me see. How through my life I have been surrounded by illness and death. Serious life-threatening illnesses in my siblings, then my mother's suicide attempts. Death hovering, desperate to help, not knowing what to do. And then training as a doctor, empowerment, tools, knowledge, a chance to protect and save lives. And then the pandemic, and that is taken away, and the people who trust me, to whom I am bound, my job, my work, as well as my spirit or—devotion—the pandemic again makes me powerless, no knowledge, no treatment—death. And now him, Dr. Hardy, whom I love, to whom I owe so much, from whom I take so much—time, space, everything. He listens and understands. How rare that is. To have a wise, brilliant, kind person listen, truly listen to me, and to understand my garbled illogical logic; my words that seem too formal and too heartfelt, both, my voice that is too soft, swallowing my words, broken by tears.

"Thank you," he says, "Your words are a gift."

His voice, resonating in my chest, holding my heart.

Later, as he does so often, Dr. Hardy has a new idea. He is—well, so often I feel utterly stuck, hopeless, trapped, the feeling of being terminally bad and inevitably wrong is overwhelming. And he has a perspective, a metaphor, a suggestion or question that—well, it's as though I have been huddled in my basement, like the crystal bowl, boxed up, and he offers an alternative way to live. Come upstairs, your exquisitely crafted house is riddled with windows, look out the front window, leaded glass, see your sycamore-lined wide street. Or look out your bedroom window-door at the enormous elm, one of the oldest trees in the neighborhood; look out your east-facing stained glass windows partially covered with vines, but letting morning light through, the sun coming over the mountains; look out from the kitchen, see the path Rockstar has made from the back door to the fence where he exchanges greetings with the neighboring dogs.

He finds a path, and we walk it together. Dr. Hardy proposes sharing the crystal bowl.

Taking turns owning, playing it. I am delighted to learn that he uses it to help other patients, people who are scared, even terrified, struggling to live, to hold on. In his words, he suggests that our joint use of it could be "our shared commitment to healing and physical regulation." And this makes it incredibly meaningful, as I do so much want to be a healer; perhaps not of hearts, the way Dr. Hardy does so expertly, but in whatever way I can. It lets me think that being small, hidden away, is not a way to avoid doing harm. To dare to think that my gift—that I have been given or can give something beautiful and healing, that the harm is in keeping it boxed away, stifled, bound, shadowed.

Meaning-ful or -less

Words, I mean. And phrases, words strewn about and slung together.

No COVID Policy.

One China Policy.

Two-State Solution.

Worldly words. Otherworldly words—

Three degrees of Glory. Third Degree. Three Degrees of Glory.

Glory to God.

God. Godliness. "Motherhood is nigh unto godliness," I heard in church, so it must be so. Or not. I am not and never will be either—god or mother. Godly or motherly. Neither.

God. Mother. Gawd, Mother. Godmother—

This, I am. My goddaughter, April, turns eight today.

Fairy godmother. Air Fairy.

I feel more moth-like, somehow.

Papery, dried-up, slightly frightening.

Moth-er. A teacher teaches, a moth-er moths?

Moth-eaten, moth balls.

Words, phrases, connections that don't connect … it is Saturday, I am not working, at least not working in clinic. It is my day to clean—well, I clean every day, but there are more required cleaning tasks on Saturday, things I have to do or I will be—something. Disreputable, shameful, sliding down the slippery slope to slovenliness. But my mind can wander with this sort of work, unlike patient care, which requires finest focus.

The word ball, mothball, leads me to then recall Rockstar, my Aussie, whom I have neglected as I endlessly clean. I seem incapable of ignoring spots on walls, wrinkles on bedspreads, pillow sham corners crushed. Sham. The other sort of sham. Shame. Shambles.

Shambala. Jambalaya. Jumbled.

Words. Schlepping about—where—? In my mind, ear, brain? And wherever they are, where am I? Here is a body, yes? Where is the mind?

Rockstar's brown eyes, slanted head, upright ear, searching upwards, for me, my look, my voice.

"Kalb," I say, Arabic for dog. "Qalb," I say, Arabic for heart. So many of my patients speak Arabic, and my attempt to learn even small pieces of the language seems to engender perhaps a bit of trust. And it is something I like to do—ask about words, learn words. Sometimes it is just a welcome dose of humor, my pronunciation is poor and sometimes the things I say sound the same, or a blend of two words. "Hello, my dog-heart. Qalb-Kabid," I say, practicing the words, sounds. Kabid is liver, I think, and can be a term of endearment. "Hello, my little liver." My dog listens and stares.

When I run, or walk, or drive somewhere or do other things, I very often listen to books. I have big headphones that keep my ears warmer and don't fall out. I look like an alien, I suppose. The books I love are wonderfully written, full of wisdom, read beautifully, and I listen again and again, because I do not listen constantly, other thoughts, words seem instead to patter along as I run. I write in my head, I plan, I look at Rockstar eying a squirrel, a yellow patch of snow, a rock. The words are there, the voice. Then I do listen and hear something new or learn something old. Then there is voice noise, beautifully wending its way with me. Not alone.

Stories. Something.

If I am trying to listen to a book, listen and hear, and realize I have missed something, I must constantly go back, again and again, until I have the exact words in my mind, no mistakes allowed. I was—or am—a bit obsessive compulsive—probably putting it that way is best.

Obsessive Compulsive Disorder, DSMV diagnosis—I am unqualified to diagnose and don't mean to be glib about an illness, and may not meet criteria, and Obsessive Compulsive Personality Disorder sounds dreadful, as any sort of Personality Disorder sounds dreadful, and obsessive compulsive tendencies or trait may be correct, but seems also shameful, and obsessive-compulsive issues makes me think of an issue of blood, or a journal, and I do not have bleeding and am not a journal, so… So this very bit of writing probably is plenty of evidence of shall we say a scrupulosity which may or may not be part of a distinct diagnosis.

"The words will always be there, you can go back if you need them," Dr. Hardy says, when I tell him I am going crazy, crazier, trying to get through a book to which I intend to listen and not able to stop hitting the backup button, listen again. Listen, self, then repeat the words—but not quite sure, back up again. A cyberspace full of words, a headspace full of words.

A full moon, when finally, I cannot ignore my dog's brown eyes and shutter the windows, blind myself to any other tasks, and go outside. The moon seems never quite full, even if the calendar says it is. Rockstar seems never quite full, and neither, perhaps, do I.

Snow White and David Whyte

David Whyte: standing with spine straight, feet slightly more than shoulder width apart, perfectly balanced, like a dancer. I watched him, then, wishing for invisibility, tried to slip without ripple into the single empty chair, no disturbance to the sound of poetry, the taut attention of the audience, the settled atmosphere of the farmhouse library.

"Welcome, Melissa," David Whyte said.

Clearly my invisible slip-in had failed.

"I am so so sorry I am late," I replied.

The room: a library or den, with straight-backed chairs in the center today, and probable permanent furniture—comfortable couches with yellow, brown, green pillows, more pillows in window seats and on the floor, alongside yoga mats. The seat I had taken, the one left, was actually a desk, the kind I had in elementary school, with the chair attached, the wooden desk with a lift-up lid and a little shelf-basket made of metal under the seat. I had tried to tuck into it, be small as a child, slip my bag beneath the seat.

We were at Bank Grounds Farm, for a week with David Whyte and the Cumbria countryside. I entered masked but saw that all the other faces were bare. They seemed naked. Too much flesh. The "guides"—four lovely men, Irish and English, who looked after us during the week—sat at a wooden table in the room adjacent. Their rough table looked made of trees—as of course it was, but as though a tree had been converted to a table with minimal human contact, the fewest necessary cuts, nails, sanding. On the tabletop: amber-colored drinks, parts of pastries, and one man's muddy boots, the legs above the boots crossed, trousers slightly muddy too. Many of the naked-faced heads were tipped back, or to one side, to rest on a wall, or the back of the couch. But none seemed sleepy: eyes were bright, fixed on David Whyte, mesmerized, alive.

I felt myself a foreigner, fresh from my life as a physician, isolated, fighting the SARS 2 coronavirus on the "front lines," to use the cliched term, of the COVID 19 pandemic. I was not working in a hospital, but in a clinic, my patients poor—Natives, homeless, refugees, elderly with co-morbidities: the people the virus kills. I myself was isolated at home, my beautiful Australian Shepherd, Rockstar, my only company. I had survived the past two-and-a-half years sheerly on walks with him, biweekly virtual visits with my psychologist, Dr. Hardy, and a fierce love of my patients, for whom I was responsible; this work was my life. I was thin, pale, usually frightened, often exhausted. And strangely shy. With a feeling of disrobing, I removed the elastic from behind my ears and slipped off my mask. I held my breath for as long as I could. Then couldn't any more.

Before my interruption, David Whyte had been telling a story of going to Skellig Michael as a young man, having saved what was, for him at the time, a great deal of money, though it was just enough to pay the ferryman. And then, when it came time—not going. Telling himself the cost, risk as solo traveler, storm…

"We hear you paid the ferryman well, have had quite a journey," he said to me that day, as I entered the room.

And it was true. A last minute flight cancellation, the world ready to travel, the airlines perhaps not so ready. Then a train strike. So, a hired car, whose driver I did indeed pay well—but having come so far, I would have honestly paid much more. It was a bit miraculous, I thought, to be just 15 minutes late for the first morning session.

Indeed, though I had left home at 6:00 AM the previous morning, and traveled across the Atlantic and across time zones, preparing for the trip had begun years earlier. Dr. Hardy had let me borrow a CD in which David Whyte speaks of beautiful questions, innocence, recites poetry—his, Mary Oliver's, Rilke's, Blake's, Wordsworth's. He also speaks of faith and Beowulf and—something in his words or his way of understanding, and his voice—well it was, to me, compelling and felt true.

Then, we both heard him speak, Dr. Hardy and I, when Whyte came to Salt Lake City. It was just after I had spent several months out of state and critically ill, in hospital. His book, *Consolations*, was one of few I had with me, there, and I read bits of it, the only thing I seemed able to read, when I was finally able to go outside, onto the wintry roof, in a wheelchair. Whyte came in February when I was home, returning to clinic work. He spoke at a Baptist church, a few blocks' walk. Soon after meeting him there, I applied to join his walking tour of the Lake District, held annually in non-pandemic times, at the end of June. I was accepted and paid my deposit. And then the COVID 19 pandemic. Travel ended. The walking tour was canceled for the next two years.

And then I had new, or newly discovered critical personal pathology, leading to evaluation and brain surgery at the Mayo clinic, then recovery from this and…

And so the 36-hour travel delay was the smallest hiccup, the last tiny bump in the road before the turn-off, the hedge-lined drive leading to the farm. I felt hidden and safe there. The hedges themselves were intricate garden art: tall, some with wild strawberries at the bottom, ivy, boxwood, flowers I didn't know, stacked upon one another. We were by a lake, Coniston Waters, upon which two swans swam, nearly always. I could see houses on the far side, cottages, and to the North, though I didn't know this until later, it flowed into the Irish

Sea. I had a single bed with a wool blanket, in a house in which the other, larger bedroom was occupied by a woman from California. We had a small bathroom with a shower, a galley kitchen and a table with a few chairs. And windows through which I watched, sketched. Landscape, water, green, gold, dark blue-grey.

Through the days, each morning, I sank into the voice, the words, rhythm, gaze, presence, poetry of the place. Each morning—each moment—felt a bit more—more okay. I suppose more calm, but also more alive. Both more real and very unreal. Was this the world? The same world where existed my patients, pandemic, my endless attempts to be tough, to work, to not fall apart? It seemed a sort of fairy tale, rather than my true-life air-fairy story. Air Fairy, Dr. Hardy's name for the way I tried to manage: no sleep, food, rest, just be tough and work. It was a strategy honed in medical school, though likely forged in childhood trauma; refined in my time as a gymnast, strengthened over and over by life—until the cracking. My own health failing. Pandemic.

Unmasked, the people with whom I spent the week: men and women, traditional aged college students through elders, from Europe, the United States, South Africa, Australia. They seemed vibrant, shiny but not in any way superficial. Whether removal from our homes, contacts, work, circumstances, or the gorgeous Cumbrian countryside, or the words of David Whyte, or the farm food, or some other magic… something burnishing was at work. I gazed in awe at beautiful strong faces, listened to voices speaking words from the heart.

There is a version of the Snow-White fairy tale I return to often. The girl, Snow White, lacks the loving gaze of a mother, has no mirror, no self, only a murderous queen stepmother, jealous and narcissistic. The child Snow White runs away and hides in a forest, surrounded by trees, animals, birds. She is helped by a hunter who kills a bear to trick the queen, sending the bear's heart rather than that of Snow

White, as proof of her death. Dwarves in a cottage become Snow White's guardians as well as her only companions. She can hide—in nature, in kindness.

I think of this, in my little cottage by the lake. No dwarves, but these kind people who, I think, would protect me. No queen, but a virus, pandemic, patients, demands, expectations. Endless work, failing to be good enough, never able to rest. A rest could be deadly for patients. There is sickness, work to be done. My white coat a privilege, a Hippocratic oath, and yet, also… I wanted to hide. I wanted a hunter's guidance, a cadre of companions, a cloak, a garden, a rest.

Later, of course, Snow White—not-dead and still most-beautiful—is known to the wicked stepmother, wicked queen. And so, disguised, the queen visits the dwarves' cottage and tricks Snow White, attempts to kill the child herself. Her first plan: an intricately sewn corset. The queen coaxes Snow White to try it on, see the beautiful ribbons, embroidery. She slips the child's arms through, turns her around, then tightens, tightens, pulling the silk strands, holding her in. Constricting and suffocating the girl. Snow White cannot breathe. Too tight. She falls over. Just in time, the dwarves get home, they undo the corset, and the child is revived.

I think of COVID. My patients who struggle to breathe. Hearing them, doing telehealth, they cough, they are scared. They do die, some, in spite of vaccines, treatment, advice. I try. I mask, tightly sealed N95 respirator, I feel I will suffocate. Gown tight. Virus. Work. Fear.

The stepmother-witch sees that again beautiful snow white, according to the magic mirror, is alive, and most fair. She again disguises herself and is let into the cottage by Snow White, this time to sell her a tortoise-shell comb, exquisitely carved. As the witch-queen uses it to comb Snow White's jet-black hair, she is poisoning her, poisoning her thoughts. I am not sure how this is deadly, but it is. Or maybe I do understand. Not good enough. Hopeless. Again, fortunately, the dwarves return to the cottage just in time to resuscitate her, somehow, perhaps by replacing the poisonous thoughts with truth, and their love.

I wonder now, here in the Lake District, if a version of this is happening. An ability to breathe and think clearly again, away from the fear, doubt, grief of pandemic medicine, the need to be tough, to work harder. It is the work I love, being a doctor, and I cannot imagine ever not doing it, as long as I am alive, nor could I imagine having been or done anything else. And it is not patients or medicine that are the corset, the comb. But something else. Toxic thoughts of self-doubt, insecurities. Medical schools that kill the tender green sprouts that were idealistic scientist humanists, eager to learn. But trained instead in self-denial. Any bodily need a weakness, any desire for rest a failing. A health care system that so often has little to do with health. A pandemic that becomes political. A black man suffocated under the knee of a white police officer, triggering protests or riots depending on one's position, but all of it poison.

Here in Coniston, hiding in the forest. With David Whyte, who asked us to call him "David." I will do so through the rest of this writing. It feels a bit informal and presumptuous, but it was his request. It's strange—he of course called me Melissa, which is my name—and rather than feeling that was too informal, I think I felt a bit shocked each time I heard it, "Melissa" in his voice. Somehow surprised that he knew my name and was speaking to me. Every time. He knows my name? He is telling me something or asking me something. Me?

In any case, David spoke of Wordsworth, naturally—we were in his hometown, or home hills. David told of a friend of the poet's youth, a somewhat shunned or unpopular boy who learned to communicate with owls, then, tragically, died at a young age.

There was a Boy

There was a Boy; ye knew him well, ye cliffs
And islands of Winander! many a time,
At evening, when the earliest stars began
To move along the edges of the hills,
Rising or setting, would he stand alone,
Beneath the trees, or by the glimmering lake;
And there, with fingers interwoven, both hands
Pressed closely palm to palm and to his mouth
Uplifted, he, as through an instrument,
Blew mimic hootings to the silent owls
That they might answer him.—And they would shout
Across the watery vale, and shout again,
Responsive to his call,—with quivering peals,
And long halloos, and screams, and echoes loud
Redoubled and redoubled; concourse wild
Of jocund din! And, when there came a pause
Of silence such as baffled his best skill:
Then, sometimes, in that silence, while he hung
Listening, a gentle shock of mild surprise
Has carried far into his heart the voice
Of mountain—torrents; or the visible scene
Would enter unawares into his mind

With all its solemn imagery, its rocks,
Its woods, and that uncertain heaven received
Into the bosom of the steady lake.

This boy was taken from his mates, and died
In childhood, ere he was full twelve years old.
Pre-eminent in beauty is the vale
Where he was born and bred: the churchyard hangs
Upon a slope above the village school;
And through that churchyard when my way has led
On summer-evenings, I believe that there
A long half hour together I have stood
Mute-looking at the grave in which he lies!

I listened to the words, thought about the meaning, but also listened to— or was inside of— the voice, rhythm, sound and breath, cadence. David Whyte wrote that beauty is the harvest of attention. And I felt the collective attention of the room. Mary Oliver wrote that attention is prayer.

Praying
It doesn't have to be
the blue iris, it could be
weeds in a vacant lot, or a few
small stones; just
pay attention.

Like all the mornings there, we listened, but also had time to speak, usually in pairs or small groups, focusing on a theme, at least at first. This is not something I do often, in real life, speak to people in this format. Or any format, beyond clinic work, occasional piano lessons, store errands, and so on. I did not know anyone there, really, but yet again they seemed more real. And perhaps there was a freedom in anonymity. And yet—many months later I remember them, and there did seem to be a closeness, or a safety there. Elizabeth spoke of her years as a psychologist, now retired but with three patients she will continue to see. I loved that, hoping Dr. Hardy will always see me. And that I can always see patients. Andre spoke of his work as a wildlife filmmaker in Australia, and his alcoholism, and what he called "my pain." He entrusted us with this, a large ruddy-faced man, sobbing. We loved him. Part of me wanted to share my own story. But I was too afraid.

I did not want to see my white coat as a corset, my medical training a poisonous combing, my work as a doctor the ultimate mask, the opacification of all mirrors. My patients did not want a vulnerable doctor, with her own needs, beliefs, ideas. They wanted, needed, competence, skill. And care and compassion, yes, but not self-care, self-compassion—care for them—my patients, work, responsibility.

When I was young, I spent time with a few girlfriends at the family cabins owned by one of their families. We swam, rode horses, rode bikes, played night games, read mystery novels, braided each other's hair, made bracelets. It felt like—maybe like one imagines childhood, and not very much like it normally is, perhaps. After I returned, and it was only a few days, really, I must have said something about enjoying it, how nice it was, or how nice they were to me. My mother told me, "They don't know you. Let's see how much they like you after they have spent more time with you, know you better."

Maybe that is it, here in England, at this farm, in this room by the lake. If they spent more time, got to know me, they would not care for me. Is that a poisonous thought? A deadly one combed in?

Each afternoon, after the reading of poetry, discussions, farmhouse lunch, we walked. The first day, we started at Kirkstone Inn, with plans to walk across St. Raven's Edge, then descend into the Troutbeck Valley. However, the rain and wind were increasingly impressive, and by the time our three Mercedes vans and David's Land Rover parked at the Inn, it was a raging storm. Edward, one of our guides who is also a publisher, skilled calligraphist, and the epitome of an English gentleman—at least in my idea of one… posture perfect, always calm. With his perfect posture and tweed cap unaffected by the gale, he stood outside our van, suggesting the rest of us stay seated inside. Edward walked towards David, who also had gotten out. No one else had, and in fact I was not sure I could, with the amount of water, the force of the wind.

I saw Edward with a hand on David's shoulder, speaking directly into his ear, both facing away from the group, toward the mountains. I think. The mountains appeared and disappeared, shrouded in storm and fog. It wasn't a long discussion, though not as brief as I'd have thought—could there be any question of us actually attempting this ascent, in this storm? Apparently so, as I later overheard David's wife thanking Edward, and both agreeing that had it been David alone, or even the two of them, David and Edward, there would have been no change in plans.

To my surprise, we did not head back to the farm, but to an alternate walk. Outside. It was beautiful and drenching and I was glad, to be out and to feel. And I was cold. We walked along Ullswater to Aira Force. Waterfalls, forests, poetry and legend. Though a sturdier path, the storm had let up only a little. I wanted to look at the fairytale trees, the hills and moving water, but mostly my head was tilted down, my focus on keeping my feet from slipping off rocks or sinking into mud. The man in front of me and the woman behind seemed to sandwich me from the wind. It was a sort of sheltering, sometimes they even held hands around me, to be sure I wasn't swept off: the man stretching his arms back, the woman reaching forward. It reminded me of playing London Bridge as a child. I felt safe. But shivered.

"Are you cold, Melissa?" David asked.

Again, the shock at my name, from him. And that he noticed. And, somehow, that it felt a bit impossible to lie.

"Um. A little. Or. Yes. But it's okay, I'm okay, it is beautiful here," I said.

He felt my poncho, which was, of course, wet. I had on five layers, some wool, some thick, the poncho, I thought, waterproof.

"This is no good. Have you got a better jacket?" I had a packable anorak sort of waterproof jacket, but was already wearing that, so I assumed it did not qualify as "better."

"Um," I said.

"Mollie," David said, not very loudly, but Mikhail, another of the lovely guides, an Irishman, was immediately at his side. David calls him Mollie, has known him since he was a boy, knows his mother as well, knew his father who died recently. I love the families, the stories, the land, clay, connections, place.

"Yes, David?" he answered.

"When we get back, take Melissa to Ambleside…" and he gave instructions for which shop, specifications for the garment to be purchased.

And I, of course, went, and bought the most resilient, weatherproof, warm jacket, in the smallest possible size. It is not eco-friendly, not recycled, as my poncho was. Nor is it organic, and neither am I sure that the working conditions of those who made it, or the energy used in its production are good, responsible. It is the best coat I have, still, for weather, cold. And somehow, being instructed to purchase it, having someone—and this someone—think that I was worth it, deserved or needed or could be of sufficient value to merit this garment—well, it meant something. Though that may be cold comfort to the exploited Chinese laborer… sigh. I hope such was not the case.

I am off track. After that first storm, we continued to have weather. Rain of course. The cook, to whom I commented on the amount of rain, said, "Welcome to Cumbria" with a great sense of pride, it seemed. But we were able to do the St. Raven's Crest the following afternoon. I drank from spring waters, while listening to David recite Gerard Manley Hopkins' "Inversnaid,"

What would the world be, once bereft

Of wet and of wildness? Let them be left,

O let them be left, wildness and wet;

Long live the weeds and the wilderness yet.

And I collected the wool of Herdwick sheep, curling white and gray and black bits that had caught on brambles and trees. I kept it, and it—along with my magnificent jacket—took up most of the space in my suitcase home.

And for some reason David's poem "The Well of Grief" ran through my head, keeping time with my footsteps, much of the afternoon.

Those who will not slip beneath
  the still surface on the well of grief,

turning down through its black water
  to the place we cannot breathe,

will never know the source from which we drink,
  the secret water, cold and clear,

nor find in the darkness glimmering,
  the small round coins,
    thrown by those who wished for something else.

That day, sadly, the pandemic also returned, or caught up to me, or I realized it was there. As it had always been, of course. Barnard, a Belgian newlywed in our group, tested positive for COVID. Though he had a negative test on arrival, as we all had, and had been vaccinated, as we all had. He and his young wife, Julia, were given separate quarters, and quarantined, meals were brought to them, they joined the morning discussions via Zoom and did not join the afternoon walks, stayed away from the rest of us. In the evenings, a masked goodnight wave from across the courtyard at the farm. Julia tested positive the next day.

And there: the pandemicky feeling that had lifted settled on me like a leaden shroud. It seemed only a matter of time before others would become ill. David and his wife had had COVID very recently, and several others in the group had had prior infections. Probably due to vaccinations, most had been mercifully mild. Relatively. In any case they didn't die, they had recovered. But much of the group had not had the virus. And some of us had sat in a van, a den, unmasked, near Barnard. Again, I realized: comfort is dangerous. Unmasking. Unknown people. Relaxing. Not paying attention. I could be contributing to the virus' ability to mutate, to continue to do harm, to become resistant to vaccinations, to the few available treatments. I could carry it to others.

But. Maybe it was just Barnard and Julia, and we had prevented it quickly and they were properly separated and not severe—just noses dripping, slight coughs. Edward went to Ambleside for paracetamol, cough drops, more rapid tests kits were searched out. The time there was so very brief. I stayed. I loved it there. Listening to David Whyte read, recite, watching swans on the lake, discovering and sitting in alcoves. I wandered, stood, watched the farmhouse work—care of the sheep, mending fences. And indoors, care of the guests, towels, linens, and the marvelous old kitchen. There were herbs and copper pots and various other things I could not name hanging from the wooden rafters.

Most in our group were coffee drinkers, but I prefer tea, and Bridgette—the young woman who brought out our food, gave us sheets and towels and shampoo—also gave me my own small metal teapot. She then let me come into the kitchen to choose my teas. She showed me where they were and said to come whenever I liked. This was a delight, the tea drunk in the alcoves, in the den, everywhere—to watch the endless chopping, boiling, kneading, roasting, steaming. The ceiling-high shelves stocked with drying herbs, spices, clean folded dishtowels. Mostly I had boiled eggs and herbal tea and noticed how beautiful the food was, hearty soups and gorgeous salads and crusty breads.

One morning our discussion included the poem "A Modest Love," by Sir Edward Dyer:

The lowest trees have tops, the ant her gall,
The fly her spleen, the little sparks their heat;
The slender hairs cast shadows, though but small
And bees have stings, although they be not great;
Seas have their source, and so have shallow springs;
And love is love, in beggars as in kings.

Where rivers smoothest run, deep are the fords;
The dial stirs, yet none perceives it move;
The firmest faith is in the fewest words;
The turtles cannot sing, and yet they love:
True hearts have eyes and ears, no tongues to speak;
They hear and see, and sigh, and then they break.

Lacking a partner, a lover, at times I despise love poems. But David spoke of a love being a work, possibly—and I do love being a doctor. And in David's voice, hearing the poem was like wandering in the hills, forest, alone, longing, but also belonging, perhaps the faces of deer, smell of acorns, even a dwarves' cottage—there is love. The poem mentions "turtles" which is a reference to turtledoves. And here I return to Snow White.

The third visit from the stepmother. She brings Snow White an apple, and when the girl takes a bite, it is ice cold in her throat and freezes her heart, then all of her. She was, it seemed, dead. Frozen. But still beautiful, her skin pale, but cheeks and lips still rosy red. The dwarves said, "We cannot bury her in the black earth," and they had a transparent glass coffin made, so she could be seen from all sides. They laid her inside, and with golden letters wrote on it her name, and that she was a princess. Then they put the coffin outside on a mountain, and one of them always stayed with it and watched over her. The animals too came and mourned for Snow White, first an owl, then a raven, and finally a dove. And the birds—emblems of wisdom, peace and love—cry. Weep for Snow White. Their tears melt the ice-maiden, and she is revived, to live in the forest with the dear dwarves, animals, trees, and far-off hunters looking out for her forever.

I sort of made up the ending, but it's a fairytale anyway, not real. And yet, I realized, here in the Lake District, the birds—Wordsworth's owl, St. Raven's Crest, Sir Edward Dyer's doves. And yet. Not careful. COVID.

One morning, someone had issued a challenge—to get into the lake, Coniston waters. Air Fairy spoke up. And I, of course, could not be wimpy, needed to prove my mettle, get into that lake. It was hardest to get to the water's edge, in a swimsuit. Of course I had layers wrapped around me, but just going out there. Shivery cold. In spite of that—if I could do this, that meant I could be tough and helpful and not harmful. So. I did. In fact, I was first in the group, wriggling out of the robe, blankets, towels, dashing into the water, quickly submerging and dashing back out and into wraps. Too cold to shriek or laugh, but still, a bit happy. Elizabeth had made a video with her phone, and since she very kindly did not post it on the site with other trip videos, What's App, I think, I was glad. It was proof. She did send it to me, individually. I think of it sometimes, these wintry days when I crawl, shriveled and shivering, out of the Crimson Lagoon lap pool. Did that really happen? The green-blue-gray and gold beauty of that place! I didn't freeze, didn't freeze into an ice-coffin maiden—in any case, not then.

The final morning discussion was held mostly outside, distanced and masked. By then six others had tested positive. All were stable, not short of breath, varying degrees of cold or flu-like symptoms. Everyone was encouraged to speak to the group. To share—something. I had known this space would be there, the invitation, and did not know what to say. I wrote to Dr. Hardy, via email. I wrote that I thought maybe I would just listen.

He wrote, "Why don't you tell them that you grew up in a constant atmosphere of hovering death and the state of terror that caused? That how as a doctor you have spent the last three years in a similar place with your very sick patients and COVID. How hard you work to keep them alive. And now how hard you are struggling to keep yourself alive."

And I did. It felt true. I would leave the next day, and so. So, I could be seen. So, I said that. I was scared, for some reason, vulnerable or disloyal somehow. But it felt true.

After I spoke, there was dead silence in the room. David Whyte, with tears in his eyes, looked at me, and thanked me.

"Thank you, Melissa. Your task now is to learn to fully inhabit your dying body. Find your voice, speak from that voice deep within yourself," he said.

That afternoon, we did not journey in the vans, enclosed and un-distanced, to a walk. The time was free for all, though for me it was Air Fairy-dictated. She had sprung the idea that I had to walk around the lake, Coniston. I thought, I have the whole afternoon, I am here on a walking tour in the Lake District, I can walk. Why not?

I started out, protein bar and vitamin water in the pockets of my great coat, as I had come to think of it—not a greatcoat, but a great coat. I had developed the lovely habit of leaving my cell phone in my room each morning. I walked and looked. I loved the hedgerows, still, looking in them for wild strawberries. And the pale green/yellow moss, sometimes fluorescent, covering trees and rocks, the way it contrasted with the fuchsia of foxgloves. I had realized on one of our group walks that the purple pink of the marathon shirt I wore under a yellowish pullover—well I was wearing these colors, of the moss and flowers. I decided it was the proper camouflage, I was blending into, becoming part of this country, the landscape. I wished or longed for that to be true.

I walked for a long time. It was the warmest it had been all week. I even pulled my arms out of my coat and tied the sleeves at my waist; I became a little worried. It had been long enough walking, then, that I did not really think I could bear walking back. So many hours. And surely… A couple passed me on bikes, then stopped to check, I thought, a map. I asked them if they knew how far it was still around the lake. They told me not too far, maybe eight miles, and also that there was a ferry up ahead, and I could take the ferry back to a point that seemed near Bank Ground Farm. So, I journeyed on. I did not see a ferry, nor did I seem to see where the lake would finally end, desperate now for that, so that I could, at last, be on the other side, headed east again, towards the farm. Instead, it seemed the lake would never end. I would look ahead, to the west, see the path seem to curve—only to realize, upon reaching that point, that it went on, the waters. And on. And on…

I stopped someone else. To my horror, this person, a fit-seeming man maybe in his twenties, a boy-man, laughed at me. I had asked how far to the end of the lake.

"It doesn't end," he said scornfully. "Or not really—it just—it just dumps into the sea."

The lake, in some form, continues until it does indeed become the

Irish Sea.

So, then my thought was the ferry. The boy-man had taken off. I did, at last, find a bridge, used by cars and tractors, which stretched across a narrow place of lake, so that I was on the north side, opposite the side of Bank Ground. I hoped that was close enough to having walked around the lake. (Close enough for what? Air Fairy?). But mostly I just wanted to get back. I asked again about a ferry, was given shrugs, I must have looked increasingly desperate and disheveled. I had long since finished my vitamin water and protein bar. Finally, in a thick York accent, an older man said "Ferry? Ferry? There's no ferry. Do you mean the gondola? There's the little gondola, but it just goes back and forth up that way, along there, back up there. For families. Where are you from?"

"Bank Ground Farms."

"Bank Ground Farms, as far as that? There's no ferry."

This said derisively, the word "ferry" with increasing incredulity.

"Do you by any chance have a phone I could use?" I asked. He did not.

Finally, a woman with two teenage children going down to the lake did let me use her cell phone. By then I was at a car park, not sure where I was, at all, along the endless shores of that lake. But the car park had a name. I was able to find a number for Bank Ground Farms and called. The cook answered.

"Hello, this is Melissa, I am one of the guests there, I am sorry to bother you, but I wonder if any of the guides is available for a moment."

"Hello," the cook in his heavy Cumbrian accent, "What's that?"

"I'm so sorry for the bother, but I need some help, I wondered if any of the guides is available? I went for a walk and I thought there was a ferry and there isn't, and I am very tired and wonder if you could get them."

"Ferry?" Again that word, with scorn. "There's no ferry," he said.

"I know," I said.

"Hang on," he said. "I don't know where the guides are, but David is here."

And before I could stop him, he was gone.

"Hello, Melissa," said David Whyte.

"HI. I am so, so sorry," I began, near tears. I explained, or tried to, what had happened, and at least was able to give him the name of the car park.

"Just a minute," he said, putting the location into his cell phone. "How did you get there?"

"I walked, but I meant to just walk back, I am sorry…"

He cut me off. "I'll be right there," he said.

And he was. I waited at the edge of the car park, along the road. I would likely have been more humiliated had I not been fully exhausted. His dark blue Land Rover bumped along the road, he got out, helped me in, and handed me a glass bottle of cold water, the best I have ever tasted.

"There's another if you need it," he said.

"Thank you," I said. "I am sorry."

"How did you get here?" he asked, as he had before.

“I walked,” I said, as I had before. “I thought I could walk around the lake but then…” trailing off.

He seemed incredulous, so I showed him my Garmin. Looking back now at that day, June 30th, 35,948 steps. Just over 16 miles.

For some reason it feels wrong to share the rest of our conversation, or maybe I just don’t want to. We did see llamas, alpacas, for which I had been on the lookout since arriving, as they are on the Bank Ground Farms website, and for which I have a fondness. They hum.

I left early the next day. By then, more than a dozen in the group had COVID. In the end, I think all who had not previously been infected got it. I rode in the front seat of a van driven by Adrien, another of the guides. He was middle aged or a bit older, carrying extra weight in his belly, with white-gray beard but otherwise balding, a ruddy complexion, and a voice like a Shakespearean actor. He did not mask. He seemed a bit sweaty, wiping his forehead and his nose frequently. He was kind, helping with my suitcases.

He seemed a bit tired, but a bit relieved, for some reason. I thanked him for the help, asked about his life. He mentioned a disabled daughter at home, and having been afraid she would get COVID and be very ill, due to her condition. However, he had just heard from his wife that the daughter had it, the week prior, and was fine, very mild symptoms. So, he Adrien, was no longer worried about it, and was quite sure that he has it. Had it. Right then, sitting unmasked beside me. He told me of all the close contact he had with infected members of the group. He wiped his nose. I rolled down my window and stayed as close to the air outside as I could.

Manchester airport and the trip home were nightmarish. I was dropped off at the wrong terminal. The lines for check-in and security snaked throughout the entire main floors of the airport.

World travelers, unmasked, bunched together. Stuck on the tarmac in the plane for over an hour, waiting for passengers to get through security, unable to leave as we had their luggage.

And many kindnesses. The large person next to me on the plane thought I looked unwell, aimed the air vents for me, at my request, got me a blanket, tried not to overhang her chair onto mine. So kind.

Rockstar, my Aussie, was at Dog Mode, where he stays when I am gone. I had arranged for grooming his final day and had to wait until evening to pick him up. It seemed impossible that I knew how to care for a dog, could manage walking, feeding, playing. I felt fairly unwell.

However, Air Fairy was there to manage me, and I went to the Crimson Lagoon to get in some running in the pool. I didn't want to have COVID. Such guilt. I should not have traveled. I needed to be back to work Monday. I didn't want to have failed, after years of pandemic. The Crimson Lagoon is huge and often I am the only person there, but definitely able to keep distant from any other swimmers. I don't swim, since having brain and spine surgery, my neck doesn't manage the motion to breathe while swimming. I don't think there are any other pool runners. In any case, I went, masked until in the pool. By that time, I was shivering and everything seemed to hurt. I could have just run in the shallower and much warmer activity pool, using my water running shoes. But. Air Fairy. Wimp. Be tough. You have to be able to do hard things and if not, then bad things will happen and… something.

I jumped—well, not really, I got into the lap pool, flotation belt in place and started running. And immediately was frozen. It seemed all muscles had turned to ice and I—had I not been in a middle lane, I would have gotten out at the side, something Air Fairy never allows. As it was, I somehow managed to propel myself along and back to the end and to crawl out. I could barely breathe, my lungs constricted, my chest corseted. The showers at the pool were cold, perpetual issues with the hot water heating system, so I sat in the hot tub/jacuzzi, shivering, then got out and piled on towels, clothes. Had I really swam—or, rather, water-run—in Lake Coniston? Did David Whyte really come to my rescue in his Land Rover? I shook my head to dry my hair a bit, not wanting to use a comb, poison thoughts. But shaking my head hurt and made me lose my balance or proprioception, so that I half-leaned, half-fell against the brick wall by my pool chair.

And I went home. It was the desert heat, the first of July, and I felt ice-cold, shivering in the sun. At my house, I got out a COVID home test, swabbing my nose, putting the drops on the card, watching as within seconds a dark purple line confirmed I had COVID. Of course. I failed. After years of pandemic. My own selfishness, taking this trip, I helped to spread the virus, helped it mutate, was now possibly responsible for some compromised person's death, or other infected person's long COVID his inability to work and loss of income and loss of ability to provide food for his family. And I also couldn't go to work myself now, leaving my patients after just having been on vacation leave.

The most despicable bit, perhaps, is that I did not regret having gone. And would do it again, it meant that much to me, and I suppose that meant, means, something very bad and wrong and selfish. I started planning for quarantine, trying to decide how long to isolate, to balance risk of transmission and laziness/should be at work, motivations, calculations, judgments. I put on my great coat, wore it as I started unpacking, cleaning, organizing. But I had to stop, truly too ill, shaking and finding it a bit hard to breath.

I needed to get Rockstar. It also felt hard to move my limbs, frozen. I felt so cold, but feverish inside. I thought of the Red Butte Gardens pond midwinter, red-orange koi visible darkly, moving beneath a foot of thick white ice. I shivered, ice-cold. But I had no raven, dove, owl to weep for and warm me. I zipped up my coat, tied the hood tightly, imagined Snow White in a forest, David Whyte in a Land Rover, and my clinic full of COVID, chaos, and patients awaiting my return.

Afterword

In the years since the COVID-19 pandemic, during which this book has slowly made its way toward publication, the experiences of being a doctor and a patient have changed. Obviously, the overwhelming number of deaths due to a new, unknown virus and the day-to-day fear and horror of trying to save my patients—this is something I hope we don't forget, but retain to be studied, not suffered.

And yet...for those who simply love their patients and want not only to "Do no harm" but to heal, ease suffering, keep patients healthy and whole—there are new obstacles, threats. Our top scientists and the medical guidelines driven by decades of outstanding research are gone, vaccine advisory panels and leadership at the CDC are comprised of politicians, not clinicians or researchers. Now my patients not only refuse additional COVID vaccinations, they question vaccines of any type, and even spurn useful, quite safe medications such as acetaminophen, no matter what the doctor they've trusted for guidance and treatment for a decade advises. My clinic now has signage and asks screening questions designed to prevent not just COVID, but measles coming into the clinic. There are such cases near the southern border, the Reservations—and now even at the local university comes an outbreak.

Technology continues its creep into the exam room. The doctors with computer screens, patients with medical knowledge from Dr. YouTube, Dr. Google, drug advertisements accompanied by Artificial Intelligence. AI is the one listening to and recording the patient's story, and even suggesting a likely diagnosis, and then ordering the evaluation and algorithmically-derived treatment. Sold as a way to free up doctors with more time for their patients and less time with electronic health record tasks, AI seems in fact designed to increase "productivity": more patients per physician, more money for the company.

I worry, still, about the patients I am not seeing—though now they are not missing due to fear of catching, or having "caught the COVID"—they fear being caught by Immigration and Customs Enforcement and being put in detention or deported. A patient tells me his green card expired two years ago, what should he do? Can I help him? I don't know, I don't think so, what should I do? Can I help him? Medicare and Medicaid funding is cut, SNAP benefits "food stamps" are cut, and patients who seem to me too ill to work at all must take second jobs to survive.

I still believe, and research clearly supports, that there is healing in the relationship between a doctor and her patients. It is possible, still, to see patients, each patient, care-fully, to use art and science to understand suffering, to use care, skill, evidence-based medicine, and love to heal. I know that the practice of medicine in this way is a gift—a gift to the doctor—work and life that have meaning. Do patients want a human doctor, with her own body's failings, her mind's biases, her ability to make mistakes—but also her willingness to hear and to love? Is there a way to make known the value of a true doctor-patient relationship, its potential to heal beyond the medicines or procedures proscribed, so that our society, increasingly focused on costs, will make it a priority, takes steps to preserve it? Are doctors with increasingly "bloody hands" willing to keep trying, or will they be ground down by the politics of increasing demands and decreasing resources, policies and cuts that harm patients and the planet? Can we, in Gandhi's words, be the change we want to see for the world, can we reverse or at least mitigate the damage done? I will hope, and I will work.

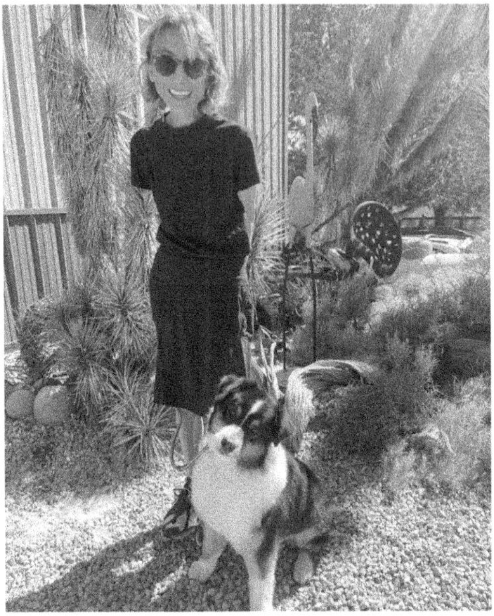

Melissa Bentley, M.D., is internal medicine physician practicing in Salt Lake City, UT, where she resides with her Australian Shepherd, Rockstar. She has additional board certification in integrative medicine, and sees patients from highly diverse backgrounds, many of whom have struggled with lack of resources, displacement from homelands, and who have had little or no consistent access to healthcare. She feels it a privilege to hear their stories, and then to be able to try to understand and diagnose illnesses, and find ways of healing, helping. Her own experiences on the other side—being a patient in a broken system of care, and struggling to forge a life of purpose and strength in spite of developmental trauma—influence her dedication to her work, as a doctor, with tools and skills to ease suffering and preserve life. Outside of clinic work, and in addition to reading and writing, she spends time running, hiking, traveling, learning, gardening, painting, playing the piano, and attending the Utah Symphony, Ballet West, and the Utah Opera—and competing in agility with Rock. She is a true nature lover and finds time outdoors with plants and animals to be healing, rejuvenating, awe-inspiring, and invaluable, and she works to preserve or restore the health of the environment she loves so that it's beauty and healing power remain in perpetuity.

www.ingramcontent.com/pod-product-compliance
Lightning Source LLC
LaVergne TN
LVHW010715061126
851857LV00014B/1193
* 9 7 8 1 6 0 4 8 9 4 2 1 9 *